MW01245097

the chakra fix

Brimming with creative inspiration, how-to projects, and useful information to enrich your everyday life, quarto.com is a favorite destination for those pursuing their interests and passions.

Inspiring | Educating | Creating | Entertaining

First published in 2022 by White Lion Publishing,
an imprint of The Quarto Group.
The Old Brewery, 6 Blundell Street
London, N7 9BH,
United Kingdom
T (0)20 7700 6700
www.quarto.com

A catalogue record for this book is available from the British Library.

ISBN 978-0-7112-6488-5
Ebook ISBN 978-0-7112-6489-2

10 9 8 7 6 5 4 3 2 1

Design by Rosamund Bird

Printed in China

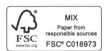

MIX
Paper from responsible sources
FSC® C016973

DISCLAIMER: The information in this book is for informational purposes only. It is not intended to diagnose, treat or prevent any illness or condition and is not a substitute for advice from a counsellor, physician, or other health care professional. There is the possibility of allergic or other adverse reactions from the use of any ingredients, essential oils or other items mentioned in this book. You should seek the advice of your doctor or other qualified health provider with any questions you may have. You should not delay seeking medical or other advice because of something you have read in this book or use the information in this book as a substitute for medication or other treatment prescribed by your medical practitioner.

The authors, editors and publisher make no representations or warranties with respect to the accuracy, completeness, fitness for a particular purpose or currency of the contents of this book and exclude all liability to the extent permitted by law for any errors or omissions and for any loss, damage or expense (whether direct or indirect) suffered by anyone relying on any infor-mation contained in this book.

the
chakra
fix

A MODERN GUIDE TO CLEANSING, BALANCING AND HEALING

Juliette Thornbury

OF LUMINOSITY CRYSTALS

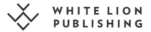

WHITE LION
PUBLISHING

CONTENTS

Introduction

Chakra healing holds immense restorative power for the mind, body and soul. It is an essential means of self-care and personal growth that nurtures our connection with ourselves and the world around us. It has taught me to stay grounded and helped me look deeper into my beliefs, thought patterns and experiences to bring me closer to my inner truth and sense of self.

My family has always had a deep connection to spiritual practices. My mother, Mallika, practices traditional kirtan, a musical form of mantra meditation, while my father, James, implemented many Buddhist practices into his life and always demonstrated the importance of meditation and maintaining a sense of spiritual awareness. After my father's passing, I became inspired to develop stronger meditation and energy healing practices, particularly through the transformative method of chakra healing. To me, finding a connection to energy through nature and subtle energy systems has become an invaluable spiritual practice.

I have worked with different forms of energy healing for more than a decade. After launching my business, Luminosity Crystals, in 2015, I became a certified crystal healer and published my first book, *The Crystal Fix*. While working with the energy of crystals, I continued to explore different avenues of spirituality and healing. I learned the importance of looking beyond the physical to determine the true source of our physical and emotional health.

Chakras are the energy centres of the body. They hold the energy of our thoughts, emotions and experiences, which influence how we think, feel and act in the present moment. Learning to recognize the beliefs and thought patterns that are holding you back is the first step in discovering how to heal yourself and move into a new state of awareness. By adjusting your ways of thinking, you can effectively align your chakras in order to live a vibrant, balanced and abundant life.

This book will provide you with the knowledge to become your own chakra healer. With a focus on practical exercises and techniques, it will expand your knowledge of energy healing, introduce you to empowering tools for self-growth and development and provide you with more than 60 chakra 'fixes' to improve your life.

I hope the advice and chakra fixes in this book will help to guide and support you through your own amazing spiritual and personal transformation, so that you can more intentionally create the life you desire.

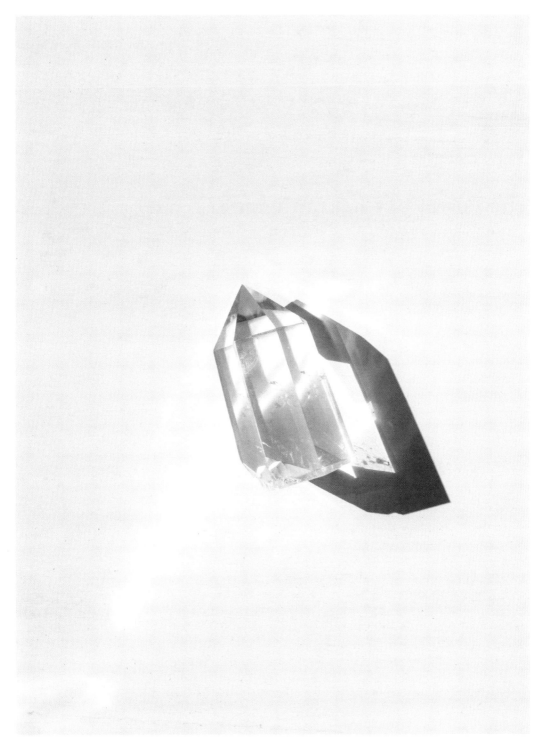

The Power of Chakra Healing

Chakra healing has ancient origins, dating back to its early traditions in India between 1500 and 500 BC, but this system of healing is as relevant today as it was then. Working with chakra energy offers the foundation to connect your mind, body and spirit. The equilibrium, health and unity that results will create a happier, healthier version of yourself.

We are made up of various energetic layers, beyond the obvious physical body. These layers are known as subtle bodies and they determine the way we process emotion and respond to life and, ultimately, define how we experience reality. There are seven subtle bodies, each extending outwards from the physical self; and these energetic layers correlate to the seven main chakras. The chakras are responsible for our different behaviours and attitudes in life. These include our sense of security, our work ethic, how we interact in our relationships and our ability to express ourselves.

Each chakra is responsible for a particular value or behaviour, such as security, love, communication and spirituality. When your chakras are aligned and working at a healthy level, you will feel a sense of harmony across all areas of your life. When a chakra is out of balance, this indicates what energy you are lacking or where you could grow and develop. For example, if you find yourself easily distracted, restless and ungrounded, this indicates an underactive root chakra.

Our actions and emotions directly affect our chakra function, just as the chakras affect our overall wellbeing. If we are feeling anxious or depressed, our basic needs are not being met, which affects our root chakra's need for safety and security. If you have gone through heartbreak or loss, you may close yourself off from others, causing your heart chakra to become underactive and making it difficult to open yourself up to new connections and experiences. If an energy centre is underactive, it can manifest as physical symptoms – for example, if you have an underactive throat chakra, you may experience throat, ear, thyroid or neck issues. Physically, illnesses are more likely to happen when your chakras are out of balance. Emotional imbalance will also occur; if your third eye chakra is underactive, you may feel disconnected from your direction in life and struggle to develop a spiritual connection.

When we work on our physical, emotional, mental and spiritual health, we strengthen our energy flow through the chakra systems. By letting go of emotional burdens, practising acceptance and forgiveness and releasing habits and thought patterns that are inhibiting your growth, you will begin to live with greater intention and develop a deeper sense of purpose.

Connecting to Your Energy Flow

Feeling the energy flow within your body can be a powerful healing experience and is an effective way to become familiar with how energy healing works. As you become more aware of the flow of energy, you will begin to feel conscious of how and where you may be directing your energy in life. The following simple exercise will allow you to activate the connection between your physical body and energy body.

Start by standing with your feet on the earth and focus on your breathing. Slowly inhale and exhale, bringing awareness to your body.

Now imagine a grounding cord pulling your energy down through your feet and into the centre of the earth. Allow this powerful earth energy to carry back up through your feet and up your spine, through to the top of your head.

Feel your body fill with this energetic light, allowing it to radiate out through the crown of your head, creating an energetic shield around your body. Visualize this stream of light returning back down through your body into the earth.

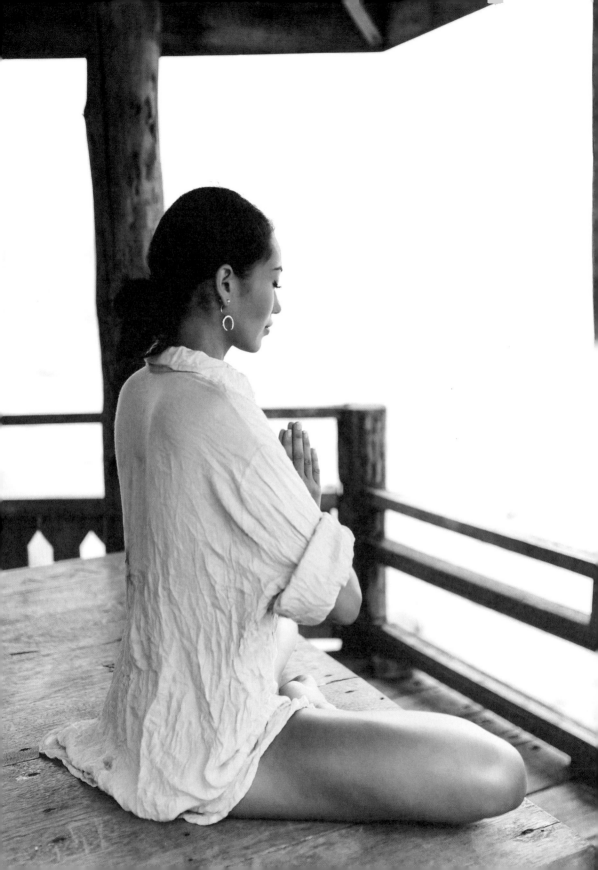

How to Use This Book

The Chakra Fix is a modern guide to chakra healing, offering a unique insight into the powerful benefits of aligning your energy centres and showing you how to implement simple techniques in practical, effective ways. Use this book as a guide to discover the physical, mental, emotional and spiritual benefits of incorporating chakra healing into your life.

Understanding the Chakras

Chapter 1 (pages 14–47) is a complete introduction to chakras and how they work to balance all the different aspects of ourselves. Each of the seven main chakras is described in detail: you will learn which energy centres are responsible for which areas of your life; you will also discover what kind of energy you need to release and what energy you need to attract more of. At the end of each section, there is advice on how to diagnose the health of that chakra, as well as how to harmonize it. Once you have worked out which of your chakras are out of balance, turn to Chapter 2 (pages 48–169) to discover the best fixes to bring them back into equilibrium.

Working with Chakras

Chapter 2 provides a deeper insight into harmonizing and restoring the individual chakras through a variety of fixes, including teas, essential oil blends, meditations, crystal grids, baths, rituals, journaling exercises and yoga poses. These step-by-step practices will help you address personal issues associated with that chakra. For example, the Crystal Grid for Connection (see page 113) will help focus your intention on healing unprocessed emotions in order to strengthen the heart chakra. And the Bath for Self-assurance (see page 132) will bring your throat chakra into alignment and promote positive self-expression, truth and open communication.

HERBS AND ESSENTIAL OILS

Herbs and essential oils can be used to activate and strengthen the energy centres of the body. The fixes in Chapter 2 include recipes for herbal teas and essential oil blends that will facilitate the healing process for the individual chakras. For the most potent plant medicine, use natural, sustainably sourced and organic ingredients.

Some essential oils may irritate sensitive skin. Prior to using an essential oil for the first time, make sure you do a patch test.

CRYSTALS AND GEMSTONES

Crystals and gemstones can be used to bring your chakras into alignment, ensuring that each energy centre is open and working at a healthy level. Chapter 2 introduces you to a selection of stones that correspond to each chakra, with advice on how to use them to support different aspects of your life. There are also crystal grids (symmetrical arrangements of stones) that you can create to balance the chakra, by directing its energy towards a specific purpose. Although clear quartz is not typically associated with most of the chakras, it acts as an energy amplifier for the other stones you will be using for each grid.

AFFIRMATIONS AND MANTRAS

Using words of affirmation, prayer or intention has a positive effect on your wellbeing and is a simple method to help you implement chakra healing in a powerful way. Chapter 2 provides examples of positive affirmations that align with each energy centre to assist you in creating positive change in your life. Mantras are sacred words or phrases often used in Hinduism and Buddhism as part of a spiritual practice. A mantra can be repeated during meditation as a way to aid focus and concentration.

RITUALS, TREATMENTS AND OTHER PRACTICES

We are constantly receiving different energy vibrations from the world around us, so it is important to cleanse our energy field regularly. By using a combination of candles, herbs, flowers, oils and crystals, it is possible to activate and heal the major energy centres of the body. Chapter 2 presents meditations, chakra balancing baths and rituals that will support your chakras and enable you to step out of your daily routine and bring greater mindfulness and connection into your life.

Chakra healing is about harmonizing all aspects of ourselves. Yoga and meditation are two of the greatest ways to achieve this. By focusing on a particular energy centre, meditation helps you to experience a stronger connection to that chakra, so that you are better able to understand its unique qualities. And by practising yoga poses specific to each chakra, you successfully embody that energy centre and begin to strengthen the connection between your mind and body. Listen to your own body as you do the yoga poses and don't push yourself beyond what feels comfortable. You should never feel pain when doing a yoga exercise.

JOURNALING

Each chakra section in Chapter 2 includes journaling questions, which you can use to work through any energetic or emotional blockages relating to your chakras. By answering these prompts honestly, you will begin to develop a greater sense of awareness; you will also discover which chakras are working at a healthy level and which are out of balance. By keeping a mindful approach to chakra healing in your day-to-day life, you will begin to experience greater wellbeing on all levels.

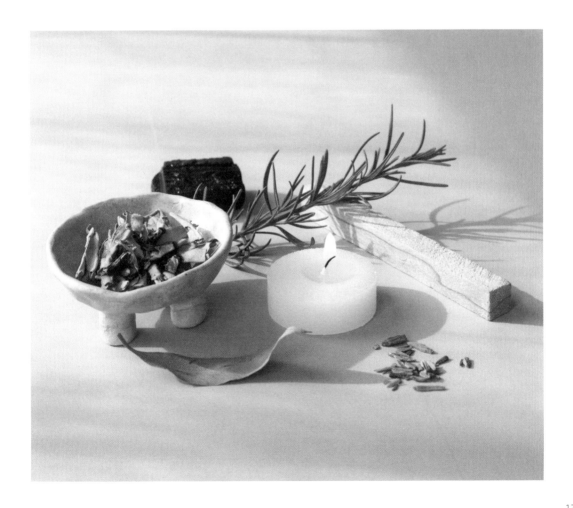

CHAPTER 1

THE CHAKRAS

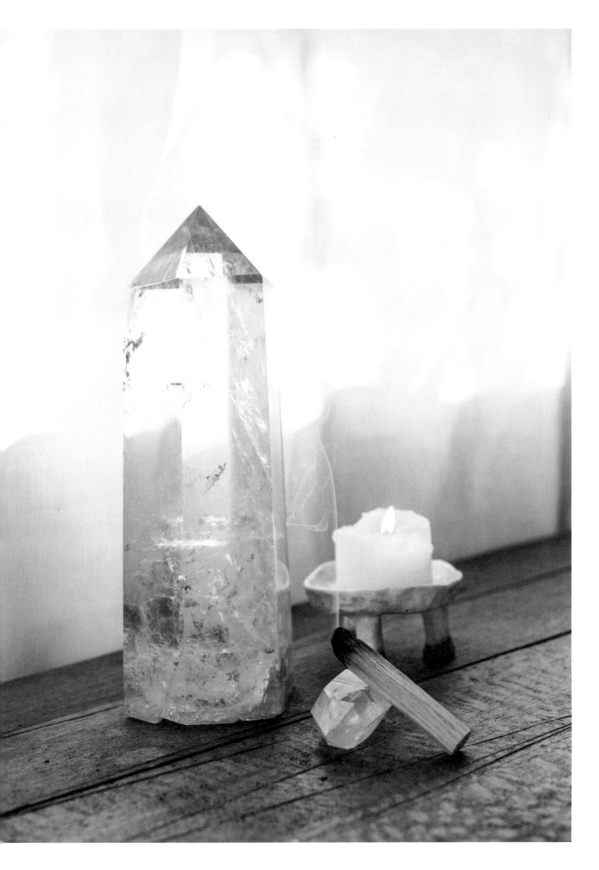

Understanding the Chakras

The word *chakra* is a Sanskrit term meaning 'spinning disc'; each chakra can be thought of as a spinning wheel of energy that acts as a major power centre for a particular aspect of your life. A lack of energy flow in the chakras causes imbalance and disconnection within the body, mind and spirit. When they are in sync, the chakras clear out stagnant energy, which helps to release emotional blockages, heal physical illness and develop a higher level of spiritual awareness. By strengthening your chakras through breathwork, meditation, yoga and other healing techniques, you are aligning your energies to achieve overall harmony.

It is believed that the chakra system originated in India when the Vedas, the oldest religious texts of India, were written. However, many Indian spiritual gurus agree that the chakra system is much older. The monks and mystics of India were masters in the art of meditation; they discovered this subtle-energy system, which was separate from, and yet connected to, their physical body. There are seven main chakras located along the spine. However, according to Sri Amit Ray, an Indian author and spiritual master, there are actually as many as 114 energy centres in the human body: seven major chakras, 21 minor chakras and 86 micro chakras. Throughout this book we will focus on the seven major chakras, which are designed to facilitate the transmission of healing energy and balance the physical, mental, emotional and spiritual energies.

The chakra system integrates both feminine and masculine energies. All beings carry both feminine (*yin*) and masculine (*yang*) energy within them. Although the chakras carry a balance of the two energies, each is associated with the gender that is being expressed in the strongest way. For example, the root chakra holds masculine energies of action, stability, determination and courage, whereas the sacral chakra holds feminine attributes of emotion, creativity, flow and intimate connection.

Each chakra also has a corresponding element. The first five are associated with the elements of earth (root), water (sacral), fire (solar plexus), air (heart) and ether (throat). The top two are connected to the elements of light (third eye) and cosmos (crown), as these two energy centres are believed to connect us beyond the earthly realm.

As we go through life, much of our reality is determined by this subtle-energy system. When we experience pain, grief, resentment or guilt, these energies reside physically within our bodies if we do not learn to process and release emotion in a healthy way. Then our chakras become underactive or completely closed, which contributes to physical and mental-health imbalances. Alternatively, when we rely too heavily on a specific chakra's energy, it can become overactive and in need of healing.

Our chakras are influenced by everything in our lives: what we do, how we think, our environment and the people close to us. These energy centres move in and out of balance naturally as we go through life's experiences. It is the chakras that hold our life-force energy, although it is our actions – and the choices we make – that keep these energies aligned or out of equilibrium. When we realign our chakras, we can heal emotional and physical illness, while also significantly increasing our overall wellbeing, relating to our health, success, relationships and spirituality.

Throughout this book you will discover effective new methods for bringing your mind, body and spirit into alignment. By working on each main energy centre, you can effectively overcome challenges in your day-to-day existence and take steps towards creating a life of happiness, abundance and wellness.

Key Chakra Terms

ENERGY

Throughout history, many cultures around the world have used the term 'energy' to describe non-physical forces in spirituality and in nature that can be felt in their own consciousness, dreams, visualizations, experiences or as an expression of a God, spiritual entity or creator.

BALANCED

If a chakra is working at the right level it is described as being balanced, healthy or active. The ideal state is for all seven chakras to be balanced and open, allowing the healthy flow of energy through the body.

UNBALANCED

If a chakra is either underactive or overactive, it is unstable and out of balance (also described as out of alignment). It needs aligning to come back to a healthy level.

OVERACTIVE

A chakra is described as overactive if it is using excessive energy and is working too hard. It needs to be brought back into alignment so that the energy is working at a healthy level.

UNDERACTIVE

A chakra is described as being underactive if it isn't as healthy or active as it should be, though not completely closed. It needs aligning or strengthening to come back to a healthy state.

CLOSED

If a chakra is no longer functioning at a healthy level or has stopped working altogether, it is described as being closed or blocked. It needs aligning or strengthening to come back to a state of wellness.

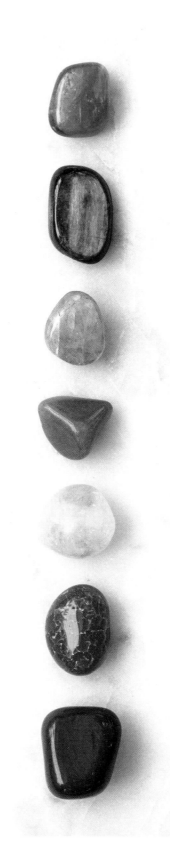

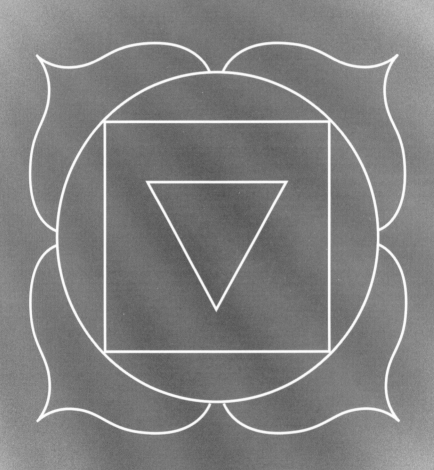

Root Chakra (*Muladhara*)

SAFETY • SECURITY • STABILITY • POWER

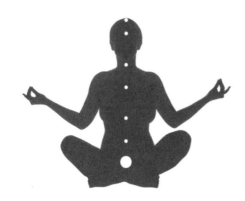

Colour	Red
Location	Base of the spine
Element	Earth
Energy	Masculine
Herbs, flowers and essential oils	Ashwagandha, black pepper, cedarwood, dandelion root, frankincense, hibiscus flowers, myrrh, patchouli, raspberry leaf, sandalwood, vetiver
Crystals and gemstones	Black tourmaline, garnet, hematite, red jasper
Mantra	Lam
Affirmations	I am safe. I am centred and grounded. I have the power to create the life I want.
Indications the chakra is balanced	You feel safe, grounded and connected to your body.
Indications the chakra is unbalanced	You feel unsafe, fearful, anxious and low in energy.

The root chakra, located at the base of the spine, is the foundation for opening the chakras above. The word *Muladhara* breaks down into two Sanskrit words: *Mula*, meaning 'root', and *Adhara*, meaning 'support' or 'base'. This energy centre houses your basic needs and instincts, including food, water, shelter and safety. The root chakra is all about empowerment and feeling strong within your body. Associated with the earth element, it establishes your physical presence in the world, allowing you to feel safe, grounded and connected to the earth. The first chakra's primary colour is red, a bold colour that is powerfully linked to vitality and survival.

The root chakra receives energy from the earth through two smaller chakras located in the feet. If we don't feel safe enough to ground ourselves and receive this nurturing earth energy, the root chakra becomes blocked. When this happens, we need to learn to address the issues that may be affecting our feelings of safety and security. How you felt during childhood is closely related to the development of your root chakra. If you felt secure in your environment while growing up, you are more likely to have your basic survival needs met as an adult, whereas if you experienced inconsistent care or traumatic events, you may find yourself with a weakened first chakra. As a result, this energy centre will need to be healed and cleared before you are able to feel safe, grounded and present in your body.

The root chakra corresponds directly to the adrenal glands, which activate the fight-or-flight response when triggered by stress or fear. In our fast-paced society, many of us are running too much adrenaline through our systems. When we are in a state of fear, we unconsciously cling to control as a way to feel safe, leaving us feeling drained and ungrounded. If our survival feels threatened, we have little energy to focus on other aspects of our lives. When the root chakra is balanced and we feel secure, we are able to be present in the moment and accepting of new opportunities. The root chakra empowers you to make the changes you need to create the life you want.

Those who embody the root chakra have a positive relationship with their physicality. Although the sacral chakra (see page 25) is the primary centre for your sexuality, it is the root chakra that powers this energy. If your root chakra is blocked, you won't feel comfortable expressing yourself openly, leading to a low sex drive and poor physical connection. People with closed root chakras also tend to struggle with setting boundaries. If you find yourself agreeing to do things purely out of obligation or find it difficult to cut yourself off from negative influences, this can indicate that you need to work on this energy centre. Once the root chakra is balanced, you are able to experience higher energy levels, a stronger work ethic and a positive attitude to life.

Diagnosing Your Root Chakra

UNDERACTIVE

If your root chakra is underactive or closed, you will feel low in energy. You may feel unsafe or fearful, making it hard for you to be happy and present in the moment. Feelings of fear, worry and anxiety are all symptoms of a closed root chakra. Physical ailments may include pain or issues related to your feet, legs and lower back, as well as poor circulation, digestion issues or reproductive problems.

BALANCED

A healthy root chakra will enable you to feel strong, grounded and safe in your body. You will feel connected to the earth, your surroundings and other people. Having a mindset of self-reliance, success and feeling motivated is another sign of a healthy root chakra.

OVERACTIVE

If the root chakra is overactive, feelings of anger, aggression and resentment are common. You may be prone to conflict and confrontation. You may also have tendencies to be overbearing or controlling towards other people.

Strategies for Balancing the Root Chakra

MEDITATION

Meditation serves as a powerful grounding tool for balancing the root chakra and will help you find strength and stability in your mind and body. As this energy centre corresponds to the earth element, try meditating outside. Focus your energy on feeling as grounded and stable as the trees around you. For a root chakra meditation, see page 58.

EXERCISE

Strengthening your physical body will nourish the root chakra too. Choose a strength-building exercise that you enjoy, such as running. Make time to nurture your physical self and build a loving relationship with your own body.

WORK

Money is one of the basic needs that is important to address so that your root chakra can heal. Set goals for your work life and learn to devote time and effort to reach your financial requirements. This will help to decrease feelings of anxiety while giving you more security to build your life.

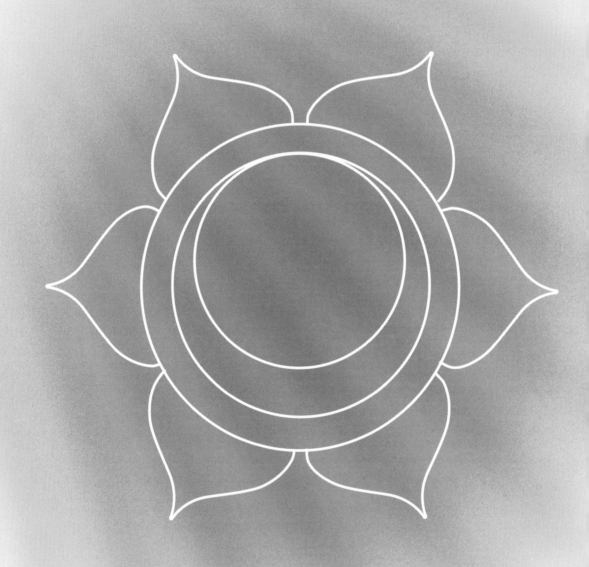

Sacral Chakra (*Svadhisthana*)

SEXUALITY • FUN • CREATIVITY • PASSION

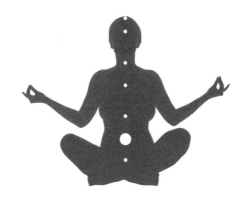

Colour	Orange
Location	Lower abdomen
Element	Water
Energy	Feminine
Herbs, flowers and essential oils	Bergamot, calendula, damiana, fennel, ginseng, mandarin, nasturtium, neroli, orange, ylang ylang
Crystals and gemstones	Carnelian, orange calcite, sunstone, tangerine quartz
Mantra	Vam
Affirmations	I am comfortable in my sexuality. I feel safe to express myself. Inspiration and creativity flow easily to me.
Indications the chakra is balanced	You feel creative, desirable and have a mentality of abundance.
Indications the chakra is unbalanced	You feel disconnected, uninspired and experience shame around your sexuality.

The sacral chakra, located 5cm (2in) below the navel, is the home of your creative, sexual and emotional energies. In Sanskrit, *Svadhisthana* means 'the dwelling place of the self'. This energy centre holds your personal power and your life-force energy. It gives you your ability to attract resources, opportunities and people into your life. Associated with the water element, it represents fluidity and versatility and provides you with the ability to flow with change. The colour of the second chakra is orange, expressing joy, vibrancy and fun.

This chakra is responsible for your emotion. It carries whatever feeling you have in your energy field, whether that is love, hate, passion or fear. An essential part of balancing your second chakra is learning to understand your emotions and how they affect your experiences and attitude to life. Consider the emotions you feel most often and which ones you have trouble processing. Being consciously aware of your emotional state is a powerful way to connect to your sacral chakra.

A balanced sacral chakra radiates warmth, bringing a sense of creativity, joy, abundance and vitality. It is centred on personal identity and is deeply connected to our partnerships with others and our relationships with the things that bring us happiness and fulfilment in life. This energy centre is all about creative expression and using your personal power to create the life you desire.

When the sacral chakra is out of balance, you may find yourself feeling overwhelmed and emotionally unstable. One of the most challenging emotions to process is shame. When we feel ashamed, it often stems from low self-esteem and low self-worth, which can be difficult to clear from the sacral chakra. Like water – the element corresponding to this chakra – our emotions move up and down in waves. This energy centre teaches us to go with the highs and lows, and to allow our sensitivity to be a part of life. The sacral chakra is a powerful tool for those who feel deeply. Learning to ground yourself and distinguish your own emotions from those of others is essential for individuals who experience high levels of empathy.

This chakra thrives on a mentality of abundance: believing that you already have enough, and that what you want to achieve is on its way to you. When your sacral chakra is balanced, you can feel this energy already available, enabling you to notice the people, opportunities and experiences that you need to help you achieve your goals.

Diagnosing Your Sacral Chakra

UNDERACTIVE

If your sacral chakra is underactive or closed, you may feel isolated and disconnected from other people. You may also be uncomfortable expressing yourself freely, and you won't feel creative. Sexual dysfunction and infertility are common physical signs of a closed sacral chakra, as well as pain in the lower back, kidneys and hips.

BALANCED

A healthy sacral chakra will have you feeling creative, desirable and connected to all life. You will be free to express yourself and develop strong, healthy relationships. Having an overall mindset of abundance and joy is another sign of a balanced sacral chakra.

OVERACTIVE

If the sacral chakra is overactive, you may struggle with setting boundaries or form unhealthy attachments, based on fear of abandonment. You may be prone to exchanging emotional or sexual energy without developing strong connections. When this energy centre becomes overactive, it can lead to substance abuse, addiction or other compulsive behaviours.

Strategies for Balancing the Sacral Chakra

MEDITATION

Meditating while focusing your attention on the sacral chakra strengthens the connection between your mind and body. Consider the version of yourself that you would like to become, and envision the life you wish to build. For a sacral chakra meditation, see page 75.

SELF-CARE

Develop a self-care ritual to help you build a loving relationship with your body. Connect to the water element by swimming in fresh water and drinking plenty of water each day. Maintaining a healthy sex life, and processing any unaddressed feelings around intimacy, is a powerful way to balance this chakra.

CREATE

Start expressing your artistic side. One of the best things you can do for your sacral chakra is to discover your imaginative talents. Try making a Tea for Creativity (see page 72) to help you connect with this energy.

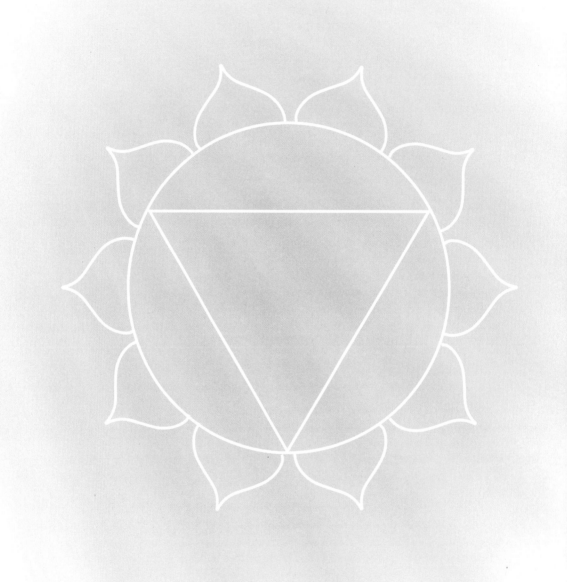

Solar Plexus Chakra (*Manipura*)

IDENTITY • CONFIDENCE • JOY • SUCCESS

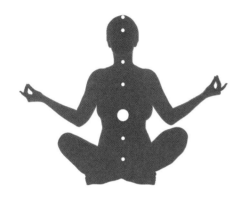

Colour	Yellow
Location	Upper abdomen
Element	Fire
Energy	Masculine
Herbs, flowers and essential oils	Chamomile, ginger, lemon, lemongrass, marshmallow root, pine
Crystals and gemstones	Citrine, pyrite, tiger's eye, topaz
Mantra	Ram
Affirmations	I am confident. I am powerful. I can achieve anything I set my mind to. I am attracting wealth and success every day.
Indications the chakra is balanced	You feel confident, motivated, joyful and self-reliant.
Indications the chakra is unbalanced	You have low self-esteem, lack of direction and find it difficult to keep motivated.

The solar plexus chakra is located near the upper abdomen and relates to your personal power, confidence and identity. In Sanskrit, *Manipura* means 'shining gem' or 'city of gems' and is the centre of who you are as a person. Associated with the fire element, this energy centre gives you a sense of purpose and motivation. It strengthens your ability to cultivate success, so that you have the confidence and willpower to achieve what you want. The colour of the third chakra is bright yellow, symbolizing warmth, optimism and happiness.

The third chakra is responsible for your self-worth, values and integrity. It projects your authentic energy out into the world, sharing what makes you unique. As we grow up, many of our values and beliefs are handed down to us by our family. These beliefs often change as we get older and discover more about ourselves and what truly resonates with us. One of this energy centre's main functions is to empower you to pursue your goals with courage. It teaches you to follow your true path, while encouraging you to master your thoughts and emotions. When we learn to overcome fear or doubt, we can develop deeper self-reliance and personal power, which profoundly impacts on the other areas of our lives.

When the solar plexus chakra is out of balance, you may lack the motivation to pursue goals and feel that you have no specific purpose in life. By strengthening this transformative energy centre, you will learn to move past your fears, enabling you to discover new opportunities for personal growth and success. When this chakra is balanced, you have a strong idea of your identity. Feeling confident enough to differentiate yourself from others is how you begin to transform into the best possible version of yourself.

The solar plexus chakra also teaches the importance of having a balanced ego. This helps you achieve your goals by giving you the confidence you need to move forward. Without this, you may lack a strong sense of identity and begin to crave validation from the outside world. Attitudes towards approval, rejection and criticism are all held in the third chakra. By balancing the solar plexus, you will find peace in your individuality.

Diagnosing Your Solar Plexus Chakra

UNDERACTIVE

If your solar plexus chakra is underactive or closed, you may find yourself craving validation from others and may lack a clear purpose. You may have low self-confidence and find it challenging to achieve your goals. Feeling helpless, insecure and unmotivated are all signs of a closed solar plexus chakra. Physical ailments may include digestion issues and eating disorders.

BALANCED

A healthy solar plexus will have you feeling confident, motivated and on the right path. You will have a strong sense of identity and won't lack willpower. Feeling secure in yourself is a sign of a balanced solar plexus chakra.

OVERACTIVE

If the solar plexus chakra is overactive, you may be opinionated, controlling or manipulative. Being overly focused on your success can mean that you neglect other areas of your life. When this energy centre becomes overactive, it may be time to reconnect with yourself and nurture other meaningful relationships.

Strategies for Balancing the Solar Plexus Chakra

MEDITATION

Meditating while focusing on the third chakra will encourage you to overcome unhealthy thought patterns and develop a stronger sense of who you are. As this chakra is associated with the fire element, try lighting a candle as part of your meditation practice. For a solar plexus meditation, see page 92.

POSITIVE HABITS

Focus on bringing fresh energy back into your life by creating healthy new habits that support your third chakra. One way to work with the fire element is by connecting with the sun; wake up early to watch the sunrise, or spend a few minutes enjoying the sunlight, and include this as a part of your daily routine.

WORK WITH GEMSTONES

Wearing or carrying topaz, tiger's eye and citrine crystals will help you cultivate a mindset of abundance. You can also hold these stones during meditation or create a Crystal Grid for Prosperity (see page 97).

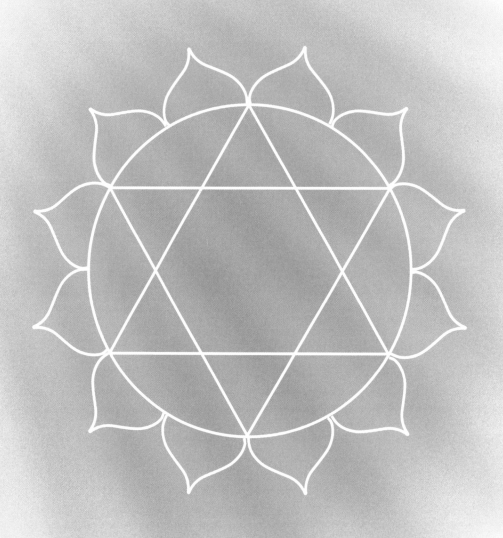

Heart Chakra (*Anahata*)

LOVE • CONNECTEDNESS • FORGIVENESS • COMPASSION

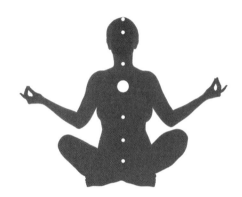

Colours	Green and pink
Location	Centre of the chest
Element	Air
Energy	Feminine
Herbs, flowers and essential oils	Hawthorn berry, hyssop, rose, rosehip
Crystals and gemstones	Emerald, green aventurine, rhodochrosite, rose quartz
Mantra	Yam
Affirmations	I choose love always. I forgive all who have wronged me. I am open to love. I have an open heart.
Indications the chakra is balanced	You feel generous, loving, forgiving and trusting of others.
Indications the chakra is unbalanced	You feel isolated and find it difficult to show love and express empathy.

The heart chakra is the fourth primary chakra in the body and is located in the centre of the chest. Represented by the air element, this energy centre can be viewed as the integration point between the upper and lower chakras, unifying the physical life with the realms of the spirit. It is the source of our most profound truths, the centre of our love, warmth and healing. It allows us to recognize the interconnectedness of all things and teaches us to live from a place of kindness and compassion. In Sanskrit, *Anahata* means 'unhurt' and is most often represented by the colour green, symbolizing health, generosity and forgiveness. When talking about self-love, sometimes a soft pink is also used, particularly in relation to crystals and gemstones.

The heart chakra governs our relationships, relating to our deep connections to others, ourselves and the universe. When this energy centre is balanced, you are naturally able to create an environment of support and empathy. Others will feel connected to your energy, drawn in by the love and acceptance you provide. When this energy is flowing freely, you are not only able to nurture your relationships with others, but also with yourself. Self-love is one of the great gifts of the heart chakra. By learning to accept and nurture yourself, you are better able to feel warm and compassionate towards others.

Your relationships are a strong reflection of the health of your heart chakra. If you feel that your relationships are weak or shallow, it can indicate that this energy centre needs healing. When we lose sight of love, compassion and empathy, our relationships suffer, disconnecting us from the people we cherish and the world around us. When the heart chakra is unbalanced, you may lack empathy and find it difficult to develop strong emotional bonds. By strengthening this energy centre, you will begin to feel a deeper connection to the world around you and discover a greater appreciation of the planet and all beings.

Forgiveness is the key to activating the fourth energy centre. We carry stress and pain within our heart chakra, and it is easy to fall into a pattern of resentment, particularly when we feel unseen or unheard. When you work on your heart chakra, it becomes easier to move forward in your relationships. Forgiving those who have wronged you in the past is perhaps one of the most effective strategies for bringing this energy centre back into balance.

Diagnosing Your Heart Chakra

UNDERACTIVE

If your heart chakra is underactive or closed, you may feel isolated, unforgiving and distrustful. Problems in relationships will also be heightened when you are emotionally closed off and uncommitted. Physically there will be a lack of energy flow from your heart to other areas of your body. Issues with the heart, lungs and respiratory system are common physical symptoms of a closed fourth chakra.

BALANCED

A healthy heart chakra will allow you to feel open and connected to the world around you. You will feel empathy and compassion towards others and have a strong sense of self-love. Feeling secure in your relationships is another sign of a healthy fourth chakra. You will be open to commitment and won't fear emotional intimacy.

OVERACTIVE

If the heart chakra is overactive, you may be prone to giving too much of your time and energy. Obsessively searching for love and not setting clear boundaries are common signs of an overactive heart chakra. You may also experience difficulties in your relationships relating to co-dependency or excessive jealousy.

Strategies for Balancing the Heart Chakra

MEDITATION

Heart chakra meditation (see page 109) is a powerful way to heal from past emotional pain. By feeling a stronger sense of peace and harmony within yourself, you are able to forgive and feel open to love and reconciliation.

SELF-LOVE

Practising self-love is an important aspect of healing your heart chakra. Create an Essential Oil Blend for Self-love (see page 108) that you can wear each day as a reminder to nurture and value yourself.

PRACTISE GRATITUDE

Make a habit of reflecting on what you are thankful for each day and then writing it down. It is entirely possible to change your perception simply by expressing gratitude for what you have.

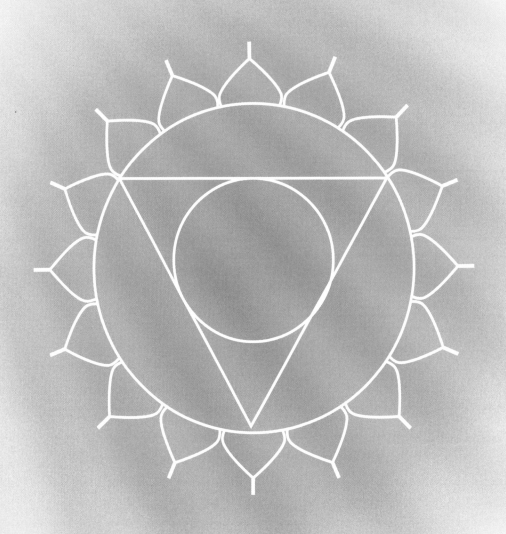

Throat Chakra (*Vishuddha*)

COMMUNICATION • UNDERSTANDING • TRUTH • EXPRESSION

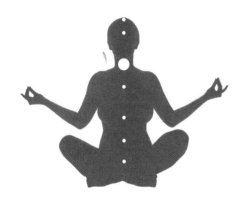

Colour	Blue
Location	Throat
Element	Ether
Energy	Masculine
Herbs, flowers and essential oils	Basil, eucalyptus, peppermint, sage, tea tree
Crystals and gemstones	Amazonite, aquamarine, hemimorphite, larimar
Mantra	Ham
Affirmations	I communicate clearly. I tell the honest truth. I speak with confidence. I live and speak my truth.
Indications the chakra is balanced	You have clear communication, speak truthfully and express yourself confidently.
Indications the chakra is unbalanced	You experience social anxiety and have difficulty expressing your thoughts and opinions.

The throat chakra is the fifth primary energy centre, represented by the colour blue, symbolizing truth and honesty. Located in the centre of the throat, it is associated with communication and self-expression. In Sanskrit, *Vishuddha* means 'especially pure' or 'to purify' and is connected to your ability to share your inner truth. This chakra is linked to the ether – the natural element that connects us to stillness, spirits and other realms. The throat chakra teaches us the power of affirmation. Through thought and communication, we have the ability to inspire and motivate, influencing how we or another person feels. By mastering the power of expression, we can transform our reality in extraordinary ways.

Think of words as if they are affirmations influencing our lives physically, emotionally and spiritually. Every word holds power and energy, which is why it is imperative to choose them wisely. Using positive affirmations raises our vibration, while negative self-talk has damaging effects on our wellbeing. When we feel restricted in the way we think, feel or speak, negative thought patterns occur, resulting in a closed or underactive throat chakra. When this energy centre is balanced, we have a healthy internal dialogue and are able to communicate our ideas with integrity. The way you express yourself in life will have a direct impact on your achievements, relationships and personal growth.

When this energy centre is blocked, you may feel socially anxious and unable to convey thoughts and emotions clearly. For some people, this can be linked to how they felt in childhood; if you grew up in an environment that didn't encourage you to express yourself openly, your throat chakra might be closed off as a result. In order to live with purpose, you must be able to communicate freely, without shame. A balanced throat chakra promotes self-expression, allowing you to share your feelings without fear of criticism. When you let go of the need to please others, you begin to experience life in a more meaningful and authentic way. Connected with the values of the heart chakra, this energy centre resonates with the energy of forgiveness and encourages the expression of love, compassion and kindness towards all.

Diagnosing Your Throat Chakra

UNDERACTIVE

When the throat chakra is underactive or closed, you may have difficulty expressing your thoughts and opinions in a constructive way. Social anxiety and insecurity around communication can be signs of an underactive fifth chakra. Physical symptoms include tension in the jaw or neck, a sore throat, thyroid problems, dental issues or earache.

BALANCED

If your throat chakra is healthy, you will be able to share your truth with ease. You will feel confident in communicating your thoughts and emotions and won't feel afraid to express yourself. Honesty and open articulation are both signs of a healthy fifth chakra.

OVERACTIVE

An overactive throat chakra will often lead people to become overbearing in their conversation style. Excessive complaining, gossiping and an aggressive tone are all signs of an overactive chakra. You may also find it difficult to allow others to express themselves or find yourself speaking without thinking.

Strategies for Balancing the Throat Chakra

MEDITATION

Meditating while focusing on the throat chakra will teach you the art of listening. Slowing the mind and focusing on your breathing encourages mindfulness; and when you are present in the moment, your true thoughts and emotions will begin to surface. For a throat chakra meditation, see page 126.

USE YOUR VOICE

Express yourself through a creative medium using your voice – whether it is writing, singing or public speaking. Sharing something positive with the world will activate the throat chakra and give you more confidence to convey your thoughts freely. For an Essential Oil Blend for Open Communication, see page 125.

JOURNALING

Keeping a journal is an effective way to transform your thoughts into words. It will help you express your ideas and desires in a constructive way, while allowing you to further reflect on your thoughts and emotions. For a throat chakra journaling exercise, see page 135.

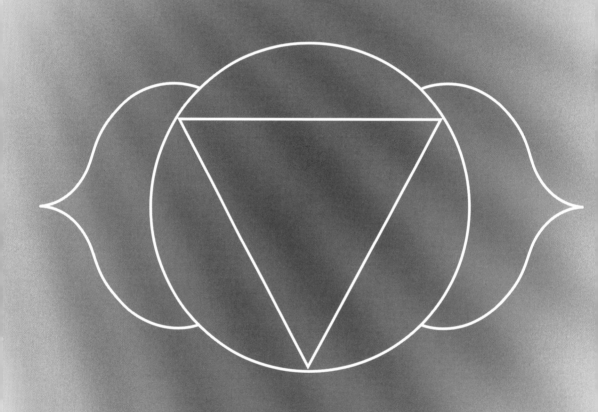

Third Eye Chakra (*Ajna*)

INSIGHT • PERCEPTION • INTUITION • INTELLECT

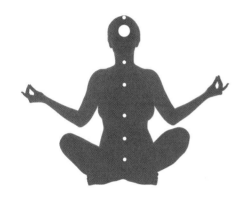

Colours	Indigo or purple
Location	Between the eyebrows
Element	Light
Energy	Feminine
Herbs, flowers and essential oils	Blue lotus, eyebright, jasmine, mugwort, passionflower, rosemary
Crystals and gemstones	Blue kyanite, labradorite, lapis lazuli, sodalite
Mantra	Sham
Affirmations	I am open to inner guidance. I am insightful and intuitive. I see and think clearly. I trust my intuition.
Indications the chakra is balanced	You have a strong sense of intuition, spiritual awareness and subtle-energy perception.
Indications the chakra is unbalanced	You lack intuition, feel confused or erratic and are unable to process thoughts clearly.

The third eye chakra, located between the eyebrows, is our centre of intuition and intellect. It governs our perception and insight and is associated with our thoughts, dreams and higher knowing. In Sanskrit, the word *Ajna* means 'perceiving'. This energy centre houses our ability to perceive the realm of subtle energies beyond our physical senses. When we quieten the mind and draw our focus inwards and away from distraction, we are able to gain further insight into our reality, while developing a deeper connection with ourselves, the universe and our surroundings. The sixth energy centre is associated with the element of light. It is most often characterized by an indigo or deep purple colour, representing the realms of spirituality and universal connection.

Connected to the pituitary gland, the third eye chakra is recognized as the centre of psychic power, spirit energies and your higher being. This is where values and beliefs are constructed and where thoughts and ideas are developed. When this chakra is open, we have a clearer perspective on the world around us. Our intuition is heightened, and we are able to better understand the complex layers of our reality. Many individuals with psychic abilities have an open third eye chakra, enabling them to experience these subtle energies and receive messages from other realms. By strengthening this energy centre, you can learn to develop your insight, enabling you to uncover new ways of seeing.

When the third eye chakra becomes overactive, it produces excess energy so that the mind becomes overly stimulated. This can make it difficult to concentrate and process knowledge and information. It is important to keep this chakra balanced in order to maintain mental clarity and feel present in the moment.

The third eye chakra relates to the subconscious and is the place from which we evaluate our beliefs and attitudes. If you find yourself replaying unhealthy thought patterns or feeling stuck in your daily routine, it may indicate that your sixth chakra needs strengthening. This energy centre teaches us to recognize our pain and fear while bravely moving forward into a new state of awareness. When the third eye chakra is closed, we have an unwillingness to address our worries and we struggle to acknowledge our true emotional state. This can lead to feelings of depression, bitterness or resentment, which can negatively affect our healing if we don't learn to process emotion in a healthy way. By working on this energy centre, we begin to strengthen our ability to embrace change, release old patterns and deconstruct limiting belief systems that no longer serve our highest good.

Diagnosing Your Third Eye Chakra

UNDERACTIVE

When this chakra is underactive or closed, you may find yourself being easily dismissive of others' opinions, overly logical or relying too heavily on your own beliefs. Experiencing narrow-mindedness and a lack of imagination are common signs of an underactive third eye chakra. Physical symptoms include headaches, depression, sleep disorders, nightmares or impaired vision.

BALANCED

When your third eye chakra is healthy, you will be able to maintain mental clarity and look beyond the mind's fears, desires and worries. This enables you to stay open to new ideas and information, leading you into a world of wisdom, knowledge and awareness. Having strong intuition and a deep sense of peace in life are also signs of a healthy sixth chakra.

OVERACTIVE

An overactive third eye chakra can lead people to become obsessed with finding 'the answer'. Excessive fantasizing or hallucinations are symptoms of an overactive sixth chakra.

Strategies for Balancing the Third Eye Chakra

MEDITATION

Practising meditation allows space for personal and spiritual transformation and encourages the development of positive thought patterns. Meditating with a focus on your sixth energy centre helps you connect to your intuition and inner guidance. For a third eye chakra meditation, see page 143.

SLEEP

Ensure you are getting enough sleep each night, ideally seven to nine hours. This energy centre is linked to lucid dreaming, astral projection and enhanced imagination; pay attention to your dreams and write them down. To strengthen your instinct, keep a record of the images you see, so that you can become familiar with new information and levels of awareness.

AROMATHERAPY

Using essential oils that correspond to this energy centre, such as blue lotus or rosemary, is a powerful way to strengthen your spiritual awareness and intuitive abilities. For an Essential Oil Blend for Clarity, see page 142.

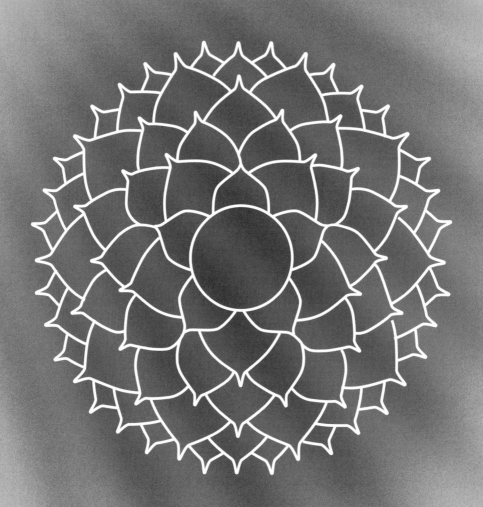

Crown Chakra (*Sahasrara*)

DIVINE GUIDANCE • CONSCIOUSNESS • SPIRITUALITY • ENLIGHTENMENT

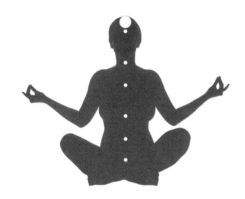

Colours	Violet or bright white
Location	Top of the head
Element	Cosmos
Energy	Feminine and masculine
Herbs, flowers and essential oils	Gotu kola, lavender, pink lotus, tulsi leaf (holy basil)
Crystals and gemstones	Amethyst, clear quartz, moonstone, selenite
Mantra	Om
Affirmations	I am connected to the universe. I seek experiences that nourish my spirit. I am at peace. I trust in divine guidance.
Indications the chakra is balanced	You experience higher awareness, have trust in the universe and maintain a peaceful mindset.
Indications the chakra is unbalanced	You lack faith and feel mentally disconnected, fearful or depressed.

Once you have a better understanding of the previous six energy centres, you will begin to feel a greater sense of peace and start to notice the energy flowing through you. The crown chakra is the energy centre of spirituality and enlightenment. Located at the top of the head and represented by a bright white or light violet colour, it is responsible for our spiritual connection to a higher power. In Sanskrit, *Sahasrara* means 'thousand-petalled lotus' and represents divinity and oneness with the universe. This energy centre is connected to the element of the cosmos, and it governs our willingness to trust in a greater intelligence to guide us on our path. Having an openness towards spirituality increases our awareness of self, others and the universe.

Associated with the pineal gland and the central nervous system, the crown chakra is responsible for the outlook that we have in life. When this energy centre is active, we feel connected to our spirituality and able to put our trust in the universe. In a society that conditions us to keep busy and on task, it can be difficult for some of us to slow down and reconnect to our higher selves. When we neglect our spiritual side, there is no room for reflection or self-growth, which is important for the health of our seventh energy centre. The crown chakra teaches us patience and stillness, and to find beauty in simplicity. It is what gives us a sense of knowing; it provides the peace and fulfilment that create a profound appreciation for all life.

The seventh energy centre enables us to connect to the realms of spirit and to trust in a higher guidance. Many of us have experienced meaningful events, synchronicities or unexplained circumstances that change our perception of life and encourage us to rethink our place in the cosmos. Connecting to the crown chakra, through signs and symbols, can help you find a way to communicate with angels or spirit guides. You may have noticed repeating numbers wherever you go, experienced profound realizations or found meaning in a particular animal encounter. Assigning significance to these unique signs is a powerful way to journey deeper and move into your spiritual power. Everything in your life is a reflection of your inner reality; staying open and receptive is the key to activating your crown chakra.

Diagnosing Your Crown Chakra

UNDERACTIVE

When the crown chakra is underactive or closed, you may feel cut off from the spirit realms, leading to a lack of purpose and direction in life. Feeling lost and without spiritual connection are common signs of a closed seventh chakra. Physical ailments include neurological disorders, depression, schizophrenia and issues relating to the brain.

BALANCED

You will have a profound connection to the universe when your crown chakra is balanced and will feel that you are being guided along the right path. You may find yourself noticing signs and synchronicities that bring you guidance. Feelings of optimism, awareness and trust are signs of a healthy crown chakra.

OVERACTIVE

When this chakra is overactive, you may feel ungrounded and unaccepting of your current physical life on earth. You may become obsessed with spirituality, to the point of neglecting your body. When the crown chakra becomes overactive, it may be time to reground your energy by spending time in nature or by focusing on your physical body, for example through yoga.

Strategies for Balancing the Third Eye Chakra

MEDITATION

Creating an environment of stillness is the most effective way to develop your connection to spirit guides and the higher realms. For a crown chakra meditation, see page 159.

AFFIRMATION AND INTENTION

Use prayer, mantras or affirmations that align with this energy centre, such as 'I am open to receiving guidance from the universe', or repeat the mantra 'Om'. Enhance this practice by visualizing a violet-white light over this energy centre and begin to notice the shift in the energy surrounding you.

BE PRESENT

Practise being present in the moment. By being mindful of where you use your time and energy, you can start to experience new ways of seeing. Practise self-care that focuses on relaxation and rejuvenation, such as a Bath for Connecting to the Universe (see page 164).

CHAPTER 2

WORKING WITH THE CHAKRAS

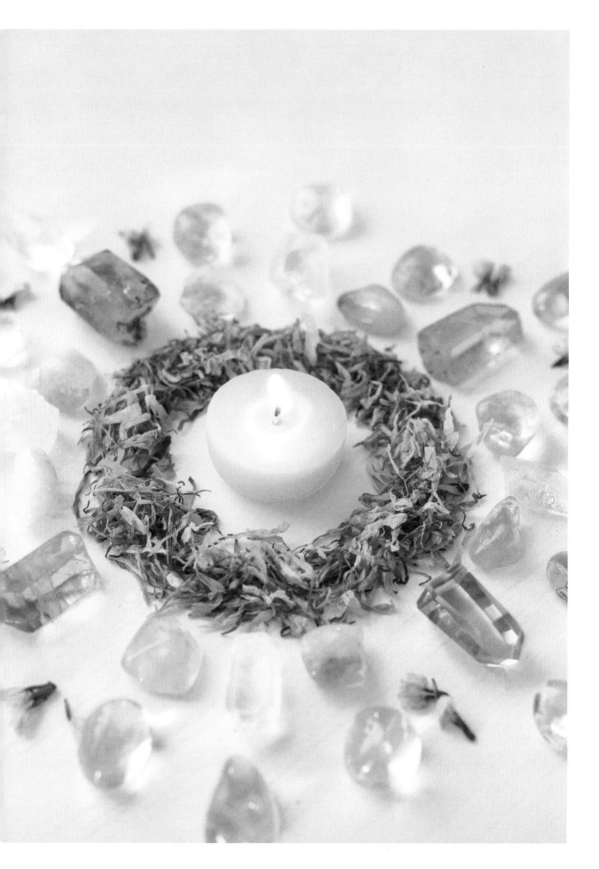

Energy Cleansing

Some of the rituals and exercises in this chapter suggest cleansing your space or an object such as a crystal. This a powerful ancient practice that has been used for centuries during sacred rituals as a way to clear stagnant or negative energy from your environment.

ENERGY CLEANSING TOOLKIT
- Sage smudge stick or palo santo wood
- Matches or lighter
- Feather (optional)
- Ceramic or glass bowl

METHOD
1   Before beginning the energy cleansing, spend a moment thinking of an intention for this practice – for example, 'I release all negativity from this space and welcome in new positive energy'.
2   Open any windows, light the sage smudge stick or palo santo wood, then blow out the flame, leaving only the smoke.
3   Cleanse the space or object:
    - **To cleanse a space**, walk clockwise around the room and use your hand or a feather to direct the smoke, ensuring that you reach all the corners of the room. Focus on your intention as you move through the space.
    - **To cleanse an object**, hold it in the smoke for a few seconds, while focusing on your intention.
4   Allow the ash to collect in the bowl and extinguish the smudge stick or palo santo wood safely after the ritual is complete.

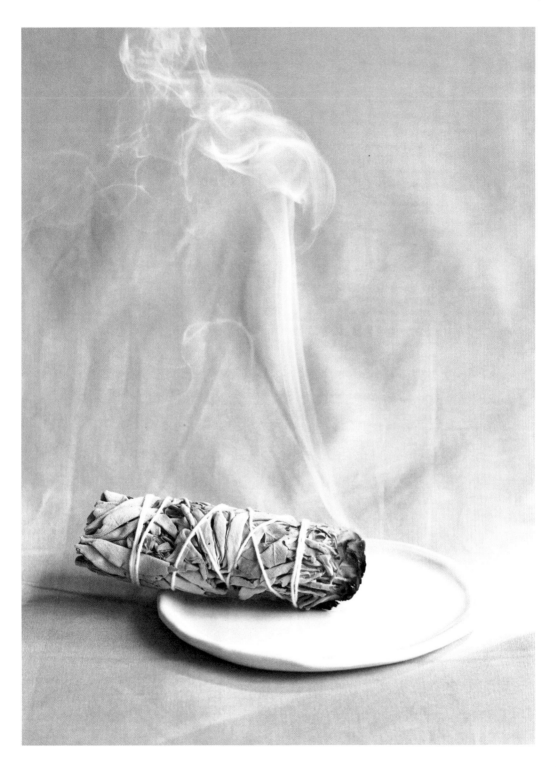

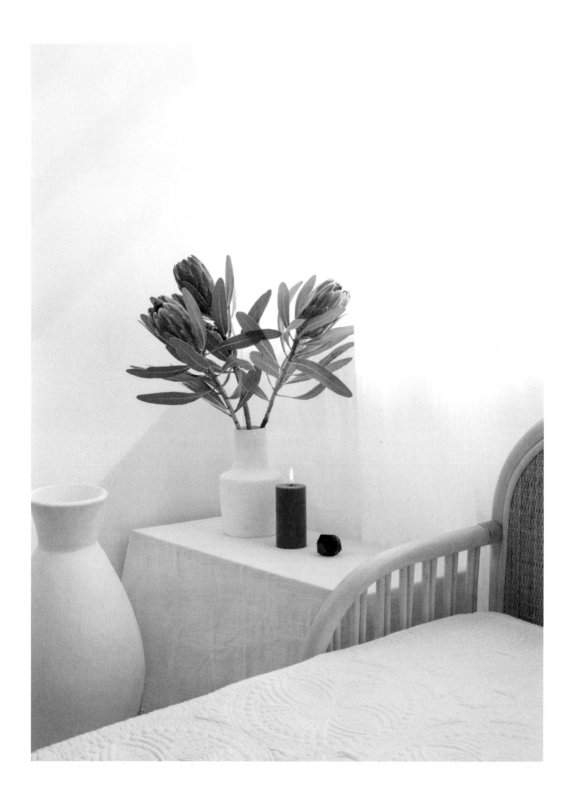

ROOT CHAKRA

ENERGY AND STABILITY

TRY THIS: For another grounding tea that will calm anxiety and help clear emotions of fear or anger, replace the hibiscus and raspberry leaves with 1 teaspoon of dried dandelion root and 1 teaspoon of dried ashwagandha root.

Tea for Grounding

Raspberry and hibiscus carry the healing properties of energy and rejuvenation. With its bold red hue, this tea activates our first chakra, promoting vitality, strength and stability. Use this infusion to balance and support your emotions, particularly when you feel mentally scattered, insecure or off-balance.

YOU WILL NEED (INGREDIENTS PER CUP)

- 1 teaspoon dried hibiscus flowers
- 1 teaspoon dried raspberry leaves
- Teapot
- 400ml (13½fl oz) boiling water
- Cup
- Sweetener of your choice (optional)

METHOD

1 Put the flowers and leaves into the teapot and pour over the boiling water.
2 Cover and leave the ingredients to steep for 5–10 minutes.
3 Pour the tea into the cup and add some sweetener, if desired.
4 Find somewhere peaceful to sit. While you drink the tea, focus on the intention of bringing balance and stability.

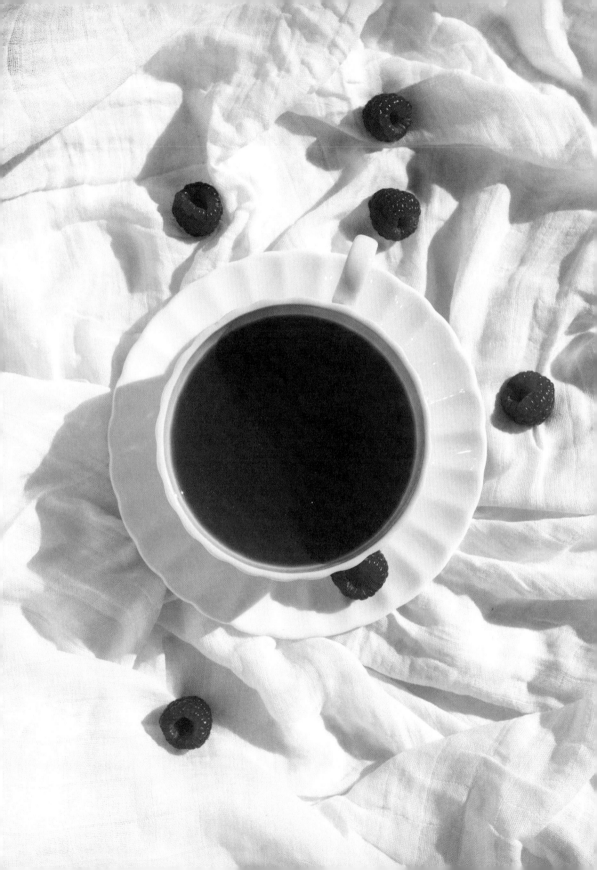

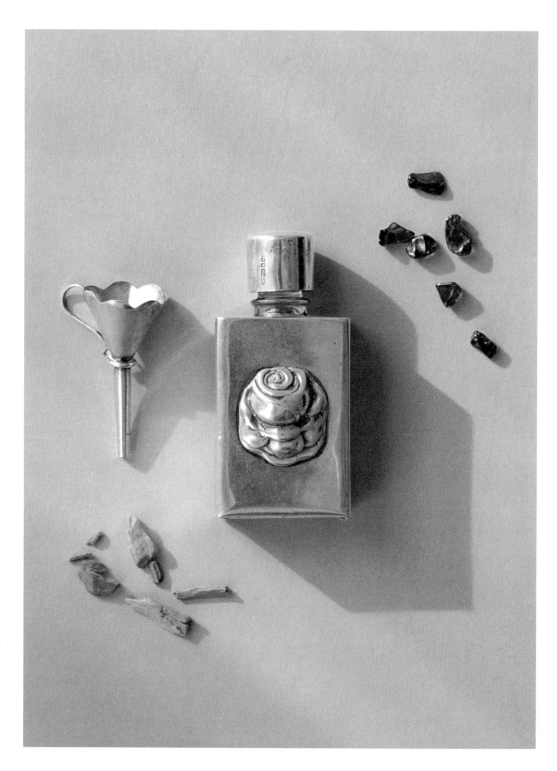

ENHANCE YOUR CHAKRA WORK:
Add a sandalwood chip or a small root chakra crystal (see page 60) to the bottle.

Essential Oil Blend for Calming the Mind

Earthy essential oils are often derived from the roots of plants, which is what contributes to their earth-like aroma, as well as their stabilizing effects. Try this essential oil blend to balance the root chakra, calm the mind and help you feel centred in times of stress or uncertainty.

YOU WILL NEED

- 4 drops vetiver essential oil
- 12 drops sandalwood essential oil
- 4 drops black pepper essential oil
- 10-ml ($\frac{1}{3}$-fl oz) glass rollerball bottle
- Small funnel or dropper
- Carrier oil, such as almond, rosehip, argan or fractionated coconut oil
- Blank label
- Pen

METHOD

1 Add the essential oils to the rollerball bottle.
2 Using a small funnel or dropper, top up the bottle with the carrier oil.
3 Insert the rollerball, close the lid and swirl to combine.
4 Write a label and stick it to the bottle.
5 To use the blend, roll a small amount on the inside of your wrists in a circular motion, or apply directly to the root chakra whenever you feel ungrounded. You can also apply it before the Meditation for Safety and Security (see page 58) to enhance the practice.

ENHANCE YOUR CHAKRA WORK:
Hold a root chakra crystal (see page 60)
in your hands during the meditation.

Meditation for Safety and Security

Designed to bring the root chakra back into alignment, this exercise will help ground and centre your energy so that you feel more present in your physical body. This meditation will also promote a sense of safety and security.

YOU WILL NEED

- Oil burner or diffuser
- Matches or lighter
- One or more root chakra essential oils (see page 21)

METHOD

1 Find a quiet, comfortable place where you can meditate with no distractions. Light the oil burner or diffuser and add the essential oils.

2 Sit in a comfortable position, with your spine straight and your shoulders relaxed. Close your eyes and take a few deep breaths, allowing your mind and body to relax completely. Feel the tension release from your face, jaw, neck and shoulders right down to your toes.

3 Now bring your focus to your root chakra, taking note of any feelings that arise. Do you feel safe and secure? Focus on feeling present in your body. Don't worry if your mind wanders; just gently bring your attention back to your breathing.

4 Visualize a red light where your root chakra resides. Imagine this glowing ball of light growing brighter with each inhale.

5 As you exhale, release any tension or stress you may be holding on to and welcome in new positive energy. Feel the aroma of the essential oils fill every cell in your body.

6 When you are ready to open your eyes, take a few deep breaths and experience a sense of presence and stillness, before bringing your awareness back to your surroundings.

7 Turn off the burner or diffuser.

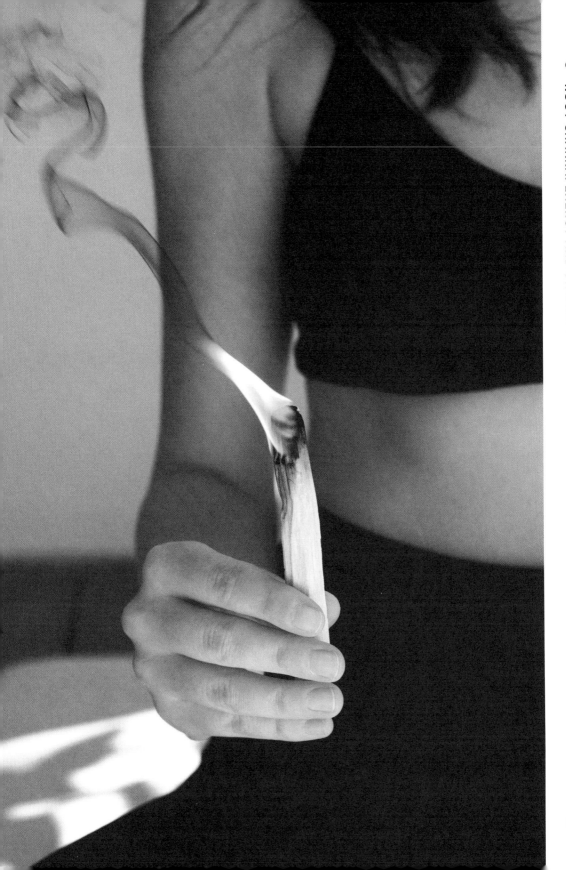

Stones for Balancing the Root Chakra

The root chakra governs our need for survival, strength and security; to balance this energy centre, consider stones that have grounding effects. These crystals can be used to enhance physical strength, as well as for grounding the physical body.

Black Tourmaline

Black tourmaline is one of the most powerful protective stones, with an exceptionally grounding energy that promotes stability and feelings of balance. It helps to eliminate tension and anxiety while increasing strength and vitality in the root chakra. With its strong cleansing abilities, black tourmaline dissipates negative energy, enhancing a peaceful and healing environment. This mystical stone has long been hailed as a powerful protective talisman by Native American peoples.

HOW TO USE THIS STONE
Keep black tourmaline by your bed to cleanse, ground and protect your energy while you sleep.

Red Jasper

With its grounding vibration, red jasper balances and restores the root chakra. Its stabilizing energy brings harmony to the mind, body and spirit. It is also known for increasing confidence, motivation, inspiration and willpower. Historically red jasper was considered a symbol of Mother Earth by Native American healers and has long been recognized as a powerful stone for enhancing physical strength and vitality.

HOW TO USE THIS STONE
Place red jasper on the body over your root chakra before bed for 20–30 minutes or longer. This will allow the stone's healing vibrations to work on this energy while having a deeply grounding effect before sleep.

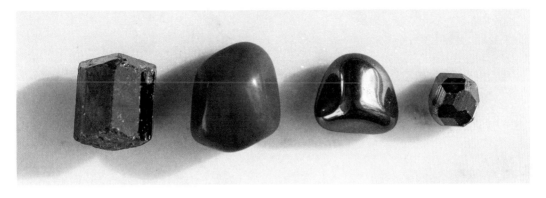

From left to right: black tourmaline, red jasper, hematite and garnet.

Hematite

Hematite is a protective and balancing stone, which brings a grounding energy that promotes harmony in the mind and the emotions. Primarily associated with the root chakra, it provides stability while encouraging a greater connection to the earth. In ancient Rome, powdered hematite was applied to the skin, as it was thought to promote strength, protection and bravery.

HOW TO USE THIS STONE
Use hematite in meditation to eliminate stress and anxiety, and to boost feelings of stability and tranquillity.

Garnet

Garnet is an effective energizing and purifying crystal, which brings emotional equilibrium, power and strength. As a root chakra stone, it enhances a profound sense of security. Garnet was believed to be a warrior's stone by the Egyptians, Greeks and Romans, who wore it as a symbol of protection, strength and bravery.

HOW TO USE THIS STONE
Wear or carry garnet to encourage self-belief and independence, and to boost a mindset of abundance, motivation and success.

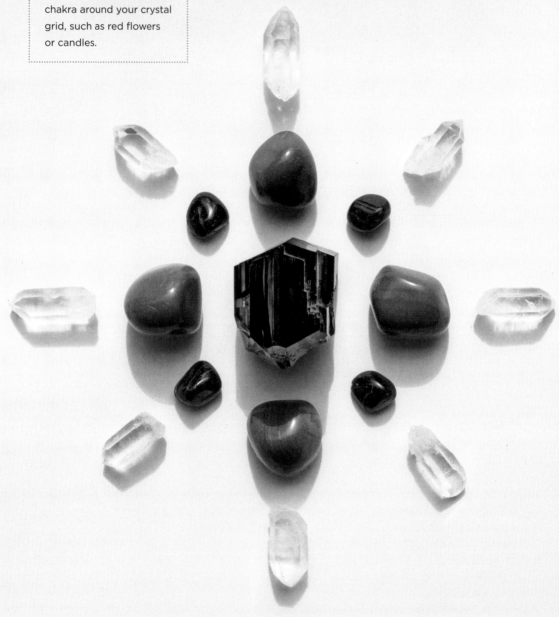

**ENHANCE YOUR
CHAKRA WORK:**
Arrange other elements
associated with the root
chakra around your crystal
grid, such as red flowers
or candles.

Crystal Grid for Stability

These crystals' grounding energies are helpful for strengthening the first chakra. Use this grid to connect your energy to the earth and help you find a stronger sense of stability and equilibrium.

YOU WILL NEED

- A clean flat surface
- Energy cleansing toolkit (see page 50)
- 1 black tourmaline
- 4 red jasper
- 4 garnet (or smaller black tourmaline)
- 8 clear quartz

METHOD

1   Decide on a flat surface to keep your grid; this should be on a table or shelf that you can revisit, but which won't be in the way of your everyday life.
2   Cleanse the crystals and the space, following the instructions on page 50.
3   Set your intention for the grid, giving the crystals a specific purpose – for example, 'I am safe', 'I welcome balance and stability into my life', 'I have the power to create the life I want'.
4   Begin creating your grid, starting with the main centre crystal; in this case, black tourmaline.
5   Add the four red jasper stones, placing one on each side of the black tourmaline.
6   Place your four garnet crystals (or smaller black tourmalines) in between the red jasper.
7   Now place each clear quartz crystal around the outside of the other stones to form a symmetrical pattern. Although it is not typically associated with the root chakra, clear quartz acts as an energy amplifier for the other stones.
8   Complete the process by focusing your energy on your intention for a minute or two. Visualize yourself feeling grounded, centred and connected to the earth.
9   Leave your grid in place for as long as you like, remembering to cleanse it occasionally and to refocus your intention.

ENHANCE YOUR CHAKRA WORK:
Add a few drops of one or two root chakra essential oils (see page 21) to the bath water.

Bath for Releasing Negativity

This bathing ritual uses grounding and energizing elements, such as hibiscus flowers and garnets, to balance the root chakra. It is ideal if you are feeling worried or fearful because it will help you find your strength and inner power.

YOU WILL NEED

- Energy cleansing toolkit (see page 50)
- Root chakra crystals (see page 60)
- Sea salt or Epsom salts
- Root chakra flowers (see page 21)
- Dandelion root, raspberry leaf or hibiscus tea
- Red beeswax or soy candles
- Calming music

METHOD

1 Cleanse the bathroom, following the instructions on page 50.
2 Run the bath, slowly adding in your healing crystals, bath salts and flowers. Add the herbal tea directly to your bath water, or save it to sip while you are bathing. Light your candles and play calming music to create a peaceful atmosphere.
3 Once you are comfortably in the bath, focus on your breathing. Close your eyes and visualize your root chakra as a bright spinning wheel of energy.
4 Let go of any tension in your body as you begin to feel centred. Choose an affirmation or intention – for example, 'I choose to feel balanced and present' – to meditate on as you release all negativity from your mind and body.
5 Extinguish the candles safely.
6 Enjoy feeling positive, centred and present as you continue your day or evening.

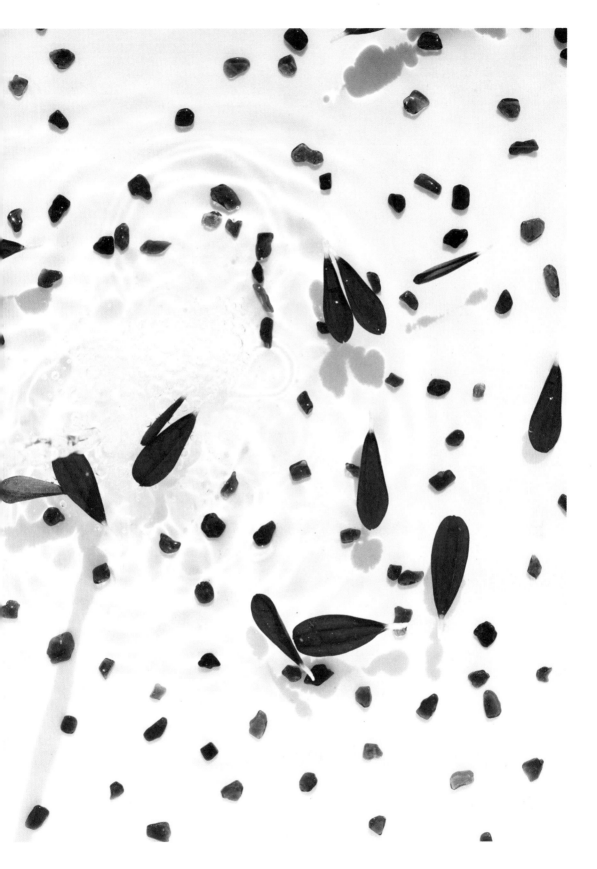

ENHANCE YOUR CHAKRA WORK:
This chakra is associated with the earth
element, so perform this ritual outside in nature.

Ritual for Energy Clearing

The root chakra is all about establishing your physical presence in the world. Try this ritual to clear stagnant energy and let go of past attachments. Although it may be difficult to process these emotions, this practice will leave you feeling lighter and more at peace with yourself.

YOU WILL NEED

- Energy cleansing toolkit (see page 50)
- Pen and paper
- One or more crystals corresponding to the root chakra (see page 60)
- Heatproof bowl
- Matches or lighter

METHOD

1 Find a quiet, comfortable place where you can meditate with no distractions. Cleanse the space, following the instructions on page 50.

2 Sit comfortably and take a few deep breaths to focus your energy. Think about what you would like to release to help you move forward; this could include old regrets, resentment or grudges that you have been holding on to.

3 Write down the things you are ready to move on from, along with a positive intention, such as 'I release what is no longer serving me' or 'I attract new and positive energy'.

4 Spend a couple of minutes meditating on your intentions while holding your crystal.

5 Focus on your root chakra and visualize a glowing red light expanding with each inhale. As you exhale, release any fear, regret or hurt you are holding on to. This will allow you to feel a greater sense of security.

6 To complete the process, place the piece of paper in the heatproof bowl and burn it, along with all you intend to release. Ensure the flames are fully extinguished when you are finished.

Root Chakra Journaling

This seven-day exercise will help you determine the health of your root chakra, while allowing you to release unprocessed emotions relating to your physical wellbeing, safety and security. Answer one of the journal prompts below each day for a week, honouring any emotions and past experiences that come up during the process.

YOU WILL NEED

- Pen and journal

METHOD

1 Begin the exercise by sitting quietly for a few minutes, focusing on your breathing to centre your energy.

2 Pick one of the following questions and answer honestly, noticing the effect it has on you:
   - Did you feel a sense of safety, stability and support as a child?
   - What does feeling grounded and connected to your body mean to you?
   - Do you feel that your needs for security are met and, if not, what steps can you take to change this?
   - Does your physical body feel strong and healthy?
   - Are you prone to feelings of anger, aggression or resentment, and do you often find yourself involved in confrontation?
   - Are there any day-to-day situations where you feel safe and grounded, and what can you do to feel more secure?
   - When in your life do you feel the most supported, connected and physically present?

3 Write your responses in your journal, working through any thoughts or emotions that arise.

4 Sit for a moment and meditate on an intention to support your root chakra – for example, 'I feel grounded and safe in my body'.

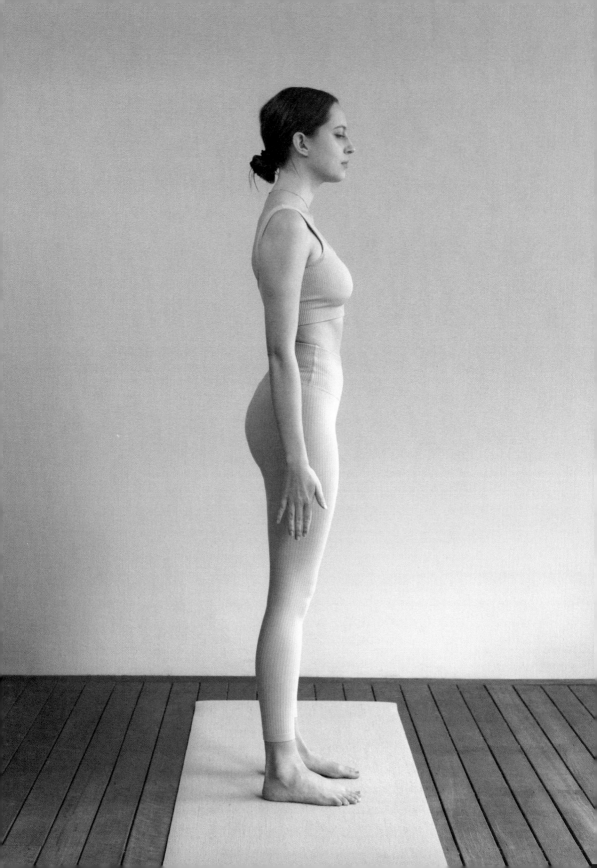

ENHANCE YOUR CHAKRA WORK:
Before you do this yoga pose, apply the Essential Oil Blend for Calming the Mind (see page 57) to your wrists or over your root chakra.

Yoga for Balance

The Mountain Pose (*Tadasana*) is associated with the earth element, allowing you to feel balanced and connected to the earth. If you are seeking stability and protection, this pose will help centre your energy and promote feelings of sanctuary and refuge.

YOU WILL NEED

- Comfortable, non-restrictive clothing
- Yoga mat

METHOD

1 Stand naturally with your feet together and your arms at your sides, palms facing forward.
2 Press your weight evenly across the four corners of your feet, engaging your thigh muscles and your core.
3 Bring your shoulders up to your ears and roll them back, so that your shoulder blades are down your back, lengthening your neck. You will feel your heart naturally lift up.
4 Gently tuck your tailbone in, to connect with and slightly lift your pelvis.
5 Take a deep breath and, as you exhale, draw your energy down through your feet.
6 Spend 3–5 breaths or longer here, feeling your energy become grounded and strong.

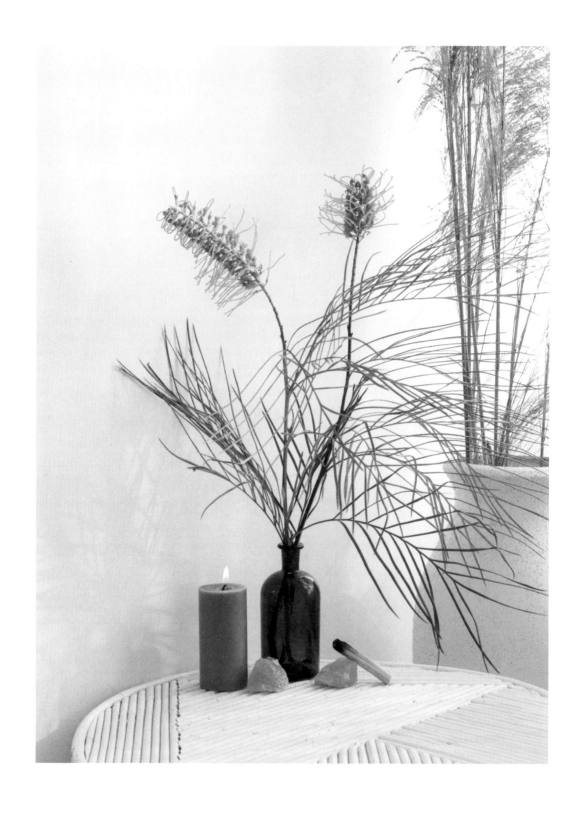

SACRAL CHAKRA

PASSION AND CREATIVITY

Tea for Creativity

The sacral chakra houses your creative, sexual and emotional energies. This powerful combination of calendula and damiana will unlock your creative energies and revitalize your imagination, particularly when you are searching for new inspiration or facing a creative block.

YOU WILL NEED (INGREDIENTS PER CUP)

- 1 teaspoon dried calendula flowers
- 1 teaspoon dried damiana leaves
- Teapot
- 400ml (13½fl oz) boiling water
- Cup
- Sweetener (optional)

METHOD

1 Put the flowers and leaves into the teapot and pour over the boiling water.
2 Cover and leave the ingredients to steep for 5–10 minutes.
3 Pour the tea into a cup and add some sweetener, if desired.
4 Sit somewhere peaceful and drink, with the intention of bringing passion and self-expression.

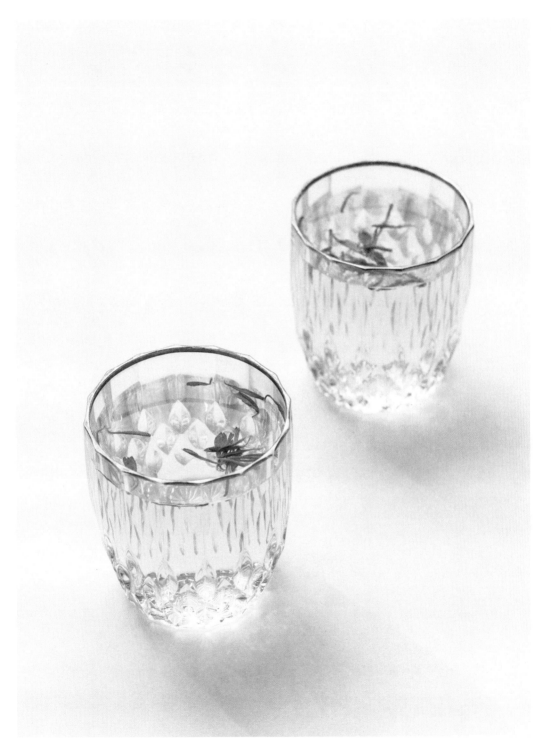

Essential Oil Blend for Vitality

Using essential oils with revitalizing and rejuvenating properties is an
effective way to balance the sacral chakra. This simple essential oil blend
will activate your second chakra, helping you feel more energized and
enhancing your sex drive.

YOU WILL NEED

- 4 drops ylang ylang essential oil
- 12 drops neroli essential oil
- 4 drops bergamot essential oil
- 10-ml (1/3-fl oz) glass rollerball bottle
- Small funnel or dropper
- Carrier oil, such as almond, rosehip, argan or fractionated coconut oil
- Blank label
- Pen

METHOD

1 Add the essential oils to the rollerball bottle.
2 Using a small funnel or dropper, top up the bottle with the carrier oil.
3 Insert the rollerball, close the lid and swirl to combine.
4 Write a label and stick it to the bottle.
5 To use the essential oil blend, roll a small amount on the inside of your
  wrists in a circular motion, or apply directly to the sacral chakra area to
  feel uplifted and energized. You can also apply it before the Meditation
  for Self-expression (see page 75) to enhance the practice.

ENHANCE YOUR CHAKRA WORK:
Hold a sacral chakra crystal (see page 76) in your hands during the meditation.

Meditation for Self-expression

This exercise is designed to alleviate feelings of insecurity and help you feel empowered to express yourself sexually, emotionally and creatively.

YOU WILL NEED

- Oil burner or diffuser
- Matches or lighter
- One or more sacral chakra essential oils (see page 25)

METHOD

1. Find a quiet, comfortable place where you can meditate with no distractions. Light the oil burner or diffuser and add the essential oils.
2. Sit in a comfortable position, with your spine straight and your shoulders relaxed. Close your eyes and take a few deep breaths, allowing your mind and body to relax completely. Feel the tension release from your face, jaw, neck and shoulders all the way down to your toes.
3. Once you are relaxed, bring your focus to your sacral chakra, taking note of any feelings that arise. Do you feel empowered and energized here or do you feel closed off and uninspired? Focus on feeling present in your body. Don't worry if your mind wanders; just gently bring your attention back to your breathing when this happens.
4. Visualize an orange light where your sacral chakra resides. Imagine this glowing ball of light growing brighter with each inhale.
5. As you exhale, release any tension or stress you may be holding on to and welcome in new inspiring energy. Feel the aroma of essential oils fill every cell in your body.
6. When you are ready to open your eyes, take a few deep breaths and experience a sense of renewed confidence and creativity before bringing awareness back to your surroundings.
7. Turn off the burner or diffuser.

Stones for Balancing the Sacral Chakra

The sacral chakra holds your personal power and life-force energy; to align this energy centre, work with stones that have energizing and creativity-boosting qualities. These crystals can be used to activate the fire within you, bringing in new empowering and self-expressive energy.

Carnelian

Carnelian enhances your courage and creative instincts and, being a high-energy stone, it enables you to feel energetic and motivated. This stone balances the sacral chakra while promoting warmth and a sense of wellbeing. When used to activate the second energy centre, carnelian also enhances sexuality and physical energy.

HOW TO USE THIS STONE
Carry carnelian to feel motivated, confident and empowered throughout your day.

Tangerine Quartz

Primarily associated with the sacral chakra, tangerine quartz is a crystal of passion, sexuality and self-expression. This stone activates the second energy centre by introducing a sense of playfulness into life. Tangerine quartz carries a warm, light energy – ideal for enhancing creativity and developing fresh ideas.

HOW TO USE THIS STONE
Wear tangerine quartz to develop a greater sense of light-heartedness and passion in relationships.

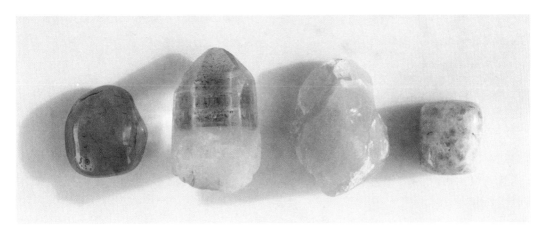

From left to right: carnelian, tangerine quartz, orange calcite and sunstone.

Orange Calcite

Orange calcite is a powerful stone when it comes to activating the sacral chakra. A highly energizing and cleansing crystal, it clears and aligns your energy so that you feel physically enlivened and open to novel experiences. It is strongly associated with physical vitality and is known to enhance both sexuality and self-expression.

HOW TO USE THIS STONE
Place orange calcite over the sacral chakra for 15–20 minutes when you first wake up, to clear energy blockages from this chakra; this will leave you feeling renewed and energized for the day ahead.

Sunstone

A bright crystal, sunstone activates and strengthens the sacral chakra. Its uplifting energy brings self-empowerment, inspiration and vivacity. The ancient Greeks believed this stone symbolized the sun god Helios, and that it conveyed courage and good luck to those who carried it. Sunstone enhances productivity, inspiration and sexuality.

HOW TO USE THIS STONE
Place sunstone over the sacral chakra during meditation and imagine its bright light activating this energy centre.

ENHANCE YOUR CHAKRA WORK: Arrange other elements associated with the sacral chakra around your crystal grid, such as orange flowers or candles.

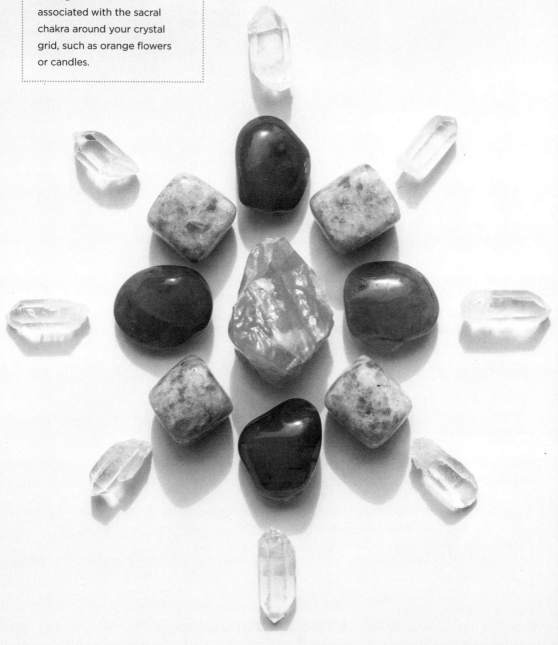

Crystal Grid for Passion and Inspiration

The crystals selected for this grid will help you to tap into your inspiration and find a refreshed sense of courage to follow your dreams.

YOU WILL NEED
- A clean flat surface
- Energy cleansing toolkit (see page 50)
- 1 orange calcite
- 4 carnelian
- 4 sunstone (or smaller orange calcite)
- 8 clear quartz (or tangerine quartz)

METHOD
1 Decide on a flat surface to keep your grid; this should be on a table or shelf that you can revisit, but which won't be in the way of your everyday life.
2 Cleanse the crystals and the space, following the instructions on page 50.
3 Set your intention for the grid, giving the crystals a specific purpose – for example, 'I feel safe to express myself' or 'Inspiration and creativity flow easily to me'.
4 Begin creating your grid, starting with the main centre crystal; in this case, orange calcite.
5 Add the four carnelian stones, placing one on each side of the orange calcite.
6 Place your four sunstone crystals (or orange calcite) in between the carnelian.
7 Now place each clear quartz (or tangerine quartz) crystal around the outside of the other stones to form a symmetrical pattern. Although it is not typically associated with the sacral chakra, clear quartz acts as an energy amplifier for the other stones.
8 Complete the process by focusing your energy on your intention for a minute or two. Visualize yourself feeling empowered, creative and full of inspiration.
9 Leave your grid in place for as long as you like, remembering to cleanse it occasionally and refocus your intention.

ENHANCE YOUR CHAKRA WORK:
Add a few drops of one or two sacral chakra
essential oils (see page 25) to the bath water.

Bath for Attracting Positive Energy

Try this powerful self-care ritual to alleviate mental fatigue and promote
emotional balance. Use warm, vibrant and energizing elements, such as
calendula flowers and carnelian crystals, to balance the second energy centre.

YOU WILL NEED

- Energy cleansing toolkit (see page 50)
- Sacral chakra crystals (see page 76)
- Sea salt or Epsom salts
- Sacral chakra flowers (see page 25)
- Calendula, ginseng or damiana tea
- Orange beeswax or soy candles
- Calming music

METHOD

1   Cleanse the bathroom, following the instructions on page 50.
2   Run the bath, slowly adding in your healing crystals, bath salts and
    flowers. Add the herbal tea directly to your bath water for extra herbal
    infusion or sip it while you are bathing. Light your candles and play
    calming music to create a peaceful atmosphere.
3   Once you are comfortably in the bath, start to focus on your breathing.
    Close your eyes and visualize your sacral chakra as a bright spinning
    wheel of energy.
4   Let go of any tension in your body as you begin to feel centred. Choose
    an affirmation or intention relating to your second chakra – for example,
    'Inspiration and creativity flow easily to me' – to meditate on as you
    attract new positive energy into your life.
5   Extinguish the candles safely.
6   Enjoy feeling vibrant, uplifted and inspired as you continue your day
    or evening.

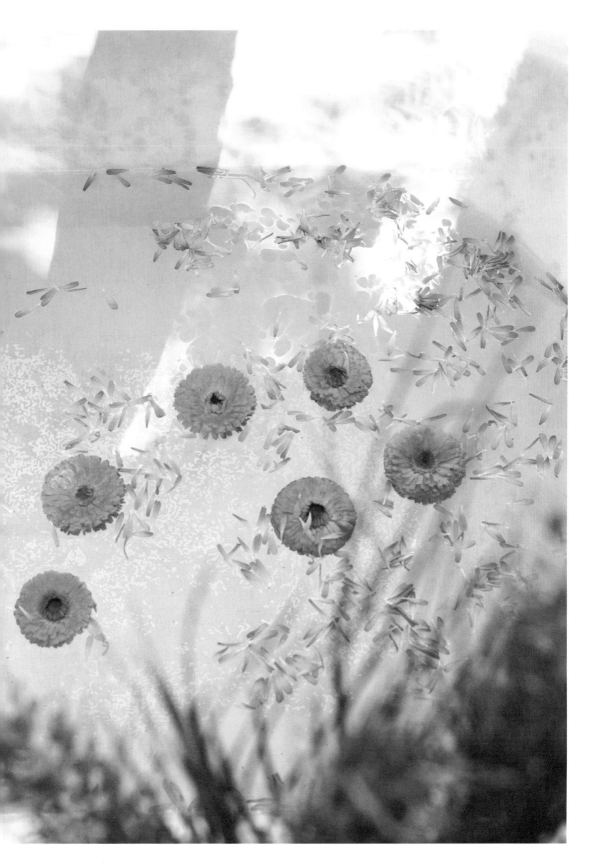

Ritual for Self-empowerment

The sacral chakra is all about developing personal power through understanding the emotions. Try this ritual to release yourself from past attachments, such as a previous unhealthy relationship you wish to let go of.

YOU WILL NEED

- Energy cleansing toolkit (see page 50)
- Pen and paper
- One or more crystals corresponding to the sacral chakra (see page 76)
- Heatproof bowl
- Matches or lighter

METHOD

1 Find a quiet, comfortable place where you can meditate with no distractions. Cleanse the space, following the instructions on page 50.

2 Sit comfortably and take a few deep breaths to focus your energy. Consider what feelings you experience most often, and which emotions you have trouble processing.

3 Write down the ideas you would like to work through and release, to help attract new energies of personal power and transformation. You may also like to write down a positive affirmation, such as 'I choose to feel courage over fear' or 'I release unhealthy attachments from my past'.

4 Spend a couple of minutes meditating on your intentions while holding your crystal.

5 Focus on your sacral chakra and visualize a glowing orange light expanding with each inhale. As you exhale, release any fear, worry or limitations you may be holding on to. This will help you heal your sacral chakra and strengthen your inner power.

6 To complete the process, place the piece of paper in the heatproof bowl and burn it, along with all you intend to release. Ensure the flames are fully extinguished when you are finished.

Sacral Chakra Journaling

This seven-day exercise will help you determine the health of your sacral chakra, while encouraging a deeper connection to your sexuality, personal power and creative energy. Answer one of the journal prompts below each day for a week, honouring any emotions and past experiences that come up during the process.

YOU WILL NEED

- Pen and journal

METHOD

1 Begin the exercise by sitting quietly for a few minutes, focusing on your breathing to centre your energy.
2 Pick one of the following questions and answer honestly, noticing the effect it has on you:
   - Do you feel creative or are you often uninspired?
   - Are you open to exploring your sexuality or do you feel closed off from this part of yourself?
   - Do you have a mentality of abundance or scarcity?
   - Which feelings do you experience most often and which do you have trouble processing?
   - Do you find it easy to feel connected with others or difficult to build meaningful relationships?
   - Do you rely on unhealthy substances or negative attachments?
   - How can you bring more fun and vibrancy into your life?
3 Write your responses in your journal, working through any thoughts or emotions that arise.
4 Sit for a moment and meditate on an intention to support your sacral chakra – for example, 'I feel inspired to express myself'.

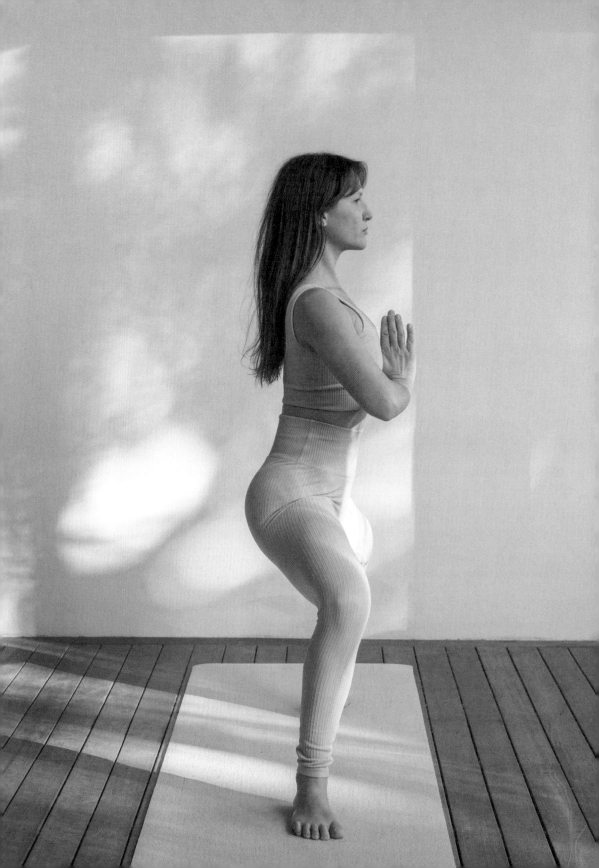

ENHANCE YOUR CHAKRA WORK:
Before you do this yoga pose, apply the
Essential Oil Blend for Vitality (see page 74)
to your wrists or over your sacral chakra.

Yoga for Personal Power

The empowering Goddess Pose (*Utkata Konasana*) opens the hips and chest
while toning the lower body. Try this pose to enhance your sense of self,
sexual energy and self-expression, particularly if you are feeling flat or
disconnected from your physical body.

YOU WILL NEED

- Comfortable, non-restrictive clothing
- Yoga mat

METHOD

1 Begin standing in Mountain Pose (see page 69) and take a breath to
centre yourself.
2 Step your feet about 1m (3ft) apart and turn your toes slightly outwards.
3 Move your hands to the centre of your chest, with the palms together.
4 Take a deep breath and, as you exhale, bend your knees directly over
your toes, so that your thighs are almost parallel to the floor (this is just
a guide; don't force this position).
5 Tuck your tailbone in slightly and press your hips forward to keep your
knees in line with your toes.
6 Keep your hands at the centre of your chest, with your shoulders down
and back. Alternatively, you may lift your hands so your upper arms are
parallel with your thighs.
7 Focus your energy into your sacral chakra and spend 3–5 breaths or
longer here.
8 Complete the exercise by stepping back into Mountain Pose.

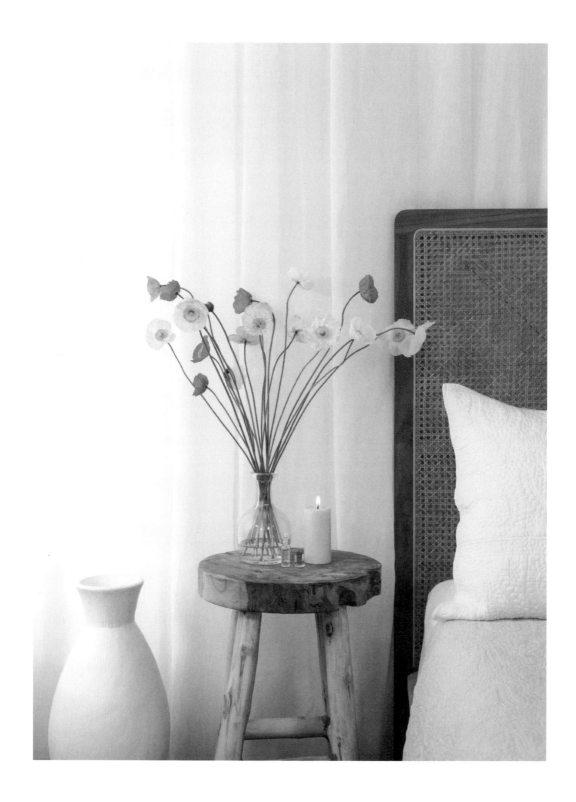

SOLAR PLEXUS CHAKRA

JOY AND SUCCESS

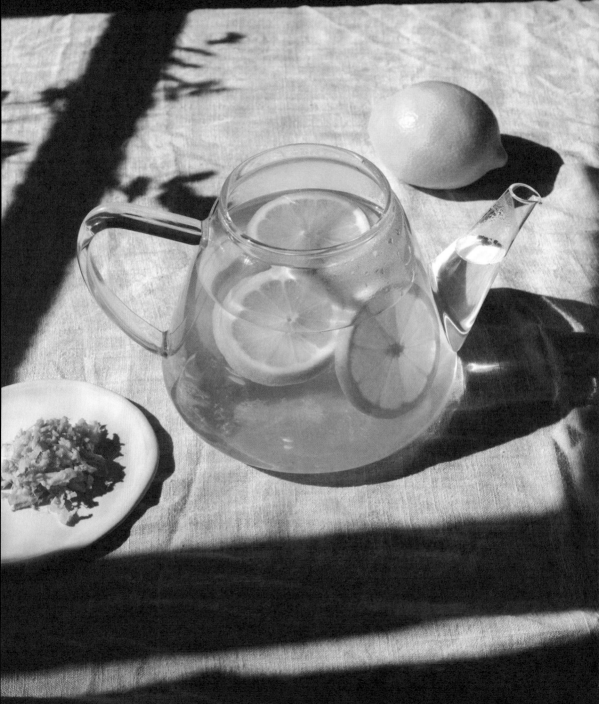

TRY THIS: For another tea that will boost your energy and lift your mood, replace the chamomile and ginger with 2 tablespoons fresh lemongrass and 1 teaspoon dried marshmallow root.

Tea for Joy

The third energy centre symbolizes warmth, optimism and happiness and corresponds to herbs and flowers carrying these properties. With its golden yellow hue, this infusion will support your solar plexus chakra, raising your spirits and revitalizing your outlook on life when you start to lose direction or face challenging times.

YOU WILL NEED (INGREDIENTS PER CUP)

- 1 teaspoon dried chamomile flowers
- 1 teaspoon fresh ginger (grated or chopped)
- 1 tablespoon fresh lemon juice or 4 slices fresh lemon
- Teapot
- 400ml (13½fl oz) boiling water
- Cup
- Sweetener of your choice (optional)

METHOD

1 Put the flowers, ginger and lemon juice or slices into the teapot and pour over the boiling water.
2 Cover and leave the ingredients to steep for 5–10 minutes.
3 Pour the tea into the cup and add some sweetener, if desired.
4 Sit somewhere peaceful. Drink the tea with the intention of bringing optimism and happiness into your life.

Essential Oil Blend for Self-confidence

Using essential oils with warming and uplifting properties is an effective way to activate your third chakra. This simple essential oil blend will help you feel more confident and energized and boost your self-esteem.

YOU WILL NEED

- 4 drops lemongrass essential oil
- 12 drops lemon essential oil
- 4 drops ginger essential oil
- 10ml ($\frac{1}{3}$-fl oz) glass rollerball bottle
- Small funnel or dropper
- Carrier oil, such as almond, rosehip, argan or fractionated coconut oil
- Blank label
- Pen

METHOD

1 Add the essential oils to the rollerball bottle.
2 Using a small funnel or dropper, top up the bottle with the carrier oil.
3 Insert the rollerball, close the lid and swirl to combine.
4 Write a label and stick it to the bottle.
5 To use the blend, roll a small amount on the inside of your wrists in a circular motion, or apply directly to the solar plexus chakra whenever you feel unmotivated or in need of a confidence boost. You can also apply it before the Meditation for Success (see page 92) to enhance the practice.

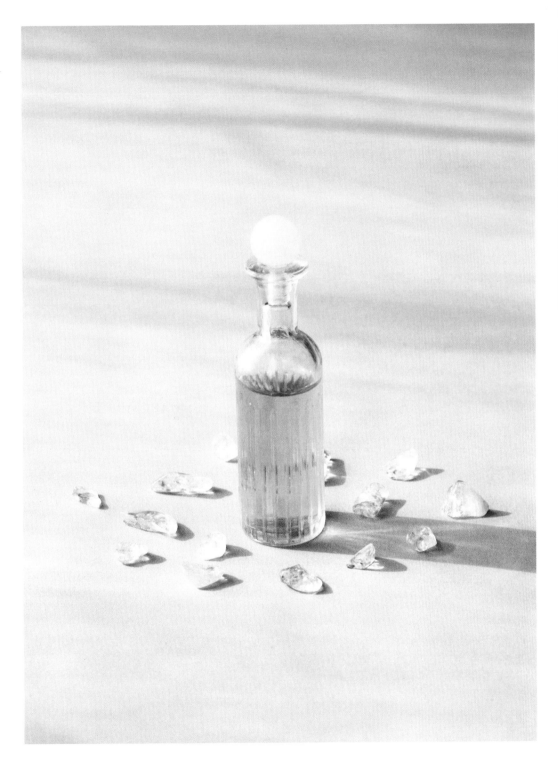

Meditation for Success

Designed to energize the solar plexus chakra, this exercise will help you develop the confidence to succeed and cultivate a mindset of abundance. Try this meditation when you lack faith in your ability to pursue your goals.

YOU WILL NEED
- Oil burner or diffuser
- Matches or lighter
- One or more solar plexus chakra essential oils (see page 29)

METHOD
1 Find a quiet, comfortable place where you can meditate with no distractions. Light the oil burner or diffuser and add the essential oils.
2 Sit in a comfortable position, with your spine straight and your shoulders relaxed. Close your eyes and take a few deep breaths, allowing your mind and body to relax completely. Feel the tension release from your face, jaw, neck and shoulders right down to your toes.
3 Now bring your focus to your solar plexus chakra, taking note of any feelings that arise. Do you feel confident, worthy and secure in yourself? Do you feel contentment or a sense of doubt? Focus on feeling present in your body. Don't worry if your mind wanders; just gently bring your attention back to your breathing.
4 Visualize a yellow light where your solar plexus chakra resides. Imagine this glowing ball of light growing brighter with each inhale.
5 As you exhale, release any self-doubt or fear you may be holding on to and welcome in new positivity. Feel the aroma of essential oils fill every cell in your body.
6 When you are ready to open your eyes, take a few deep breaths and experience a sense of self-belief and inner power, before bringing awareness back to your surroundings.
7 Turn off the burner or diffuser.

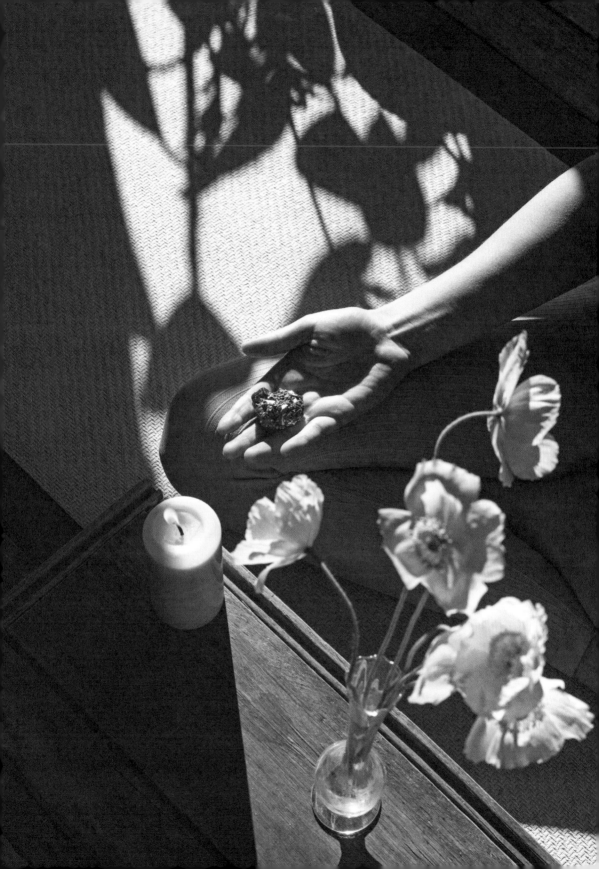

Stones for Balancing the Solar Plexus Chakra

The solar plexus chakra is responsible for your confidence, identity and who you are as a person; to balance the fire energy of this centre, consider stones that carry uplifting and empowering qualities. Use these crystals to cultivate a mindset of abundance and to bring revitalizing energy into your life.

Pyrite

Pyrite carries strong energies of personal power and happiness. Known as an effective manifestation stone, it activates the solar plexus chakra by amplifying energies of plenty and success. This crystal also reduces mental fatigue and enhances feelings of innate power and determination, while promoting personal development.

HOW TO USE THIS STONE
Keep pyrite in your office or workspace to cultivate the energy of abundance and success.

Citrine

With its vibrant energy, citrine is known for its ability to attract happiness and prosperity. Primarily associated with the solar plexus chakra, this stone magnifies your ability to manifest abundance and joy, while enhancing the energies of productivity and inspiration. Historically, this crystal was worn to attract wealth and victory.

HOW TO USE THIS STONE
Wear citrine to benefit from its uplifting, radiant energies and to protect against negativity.

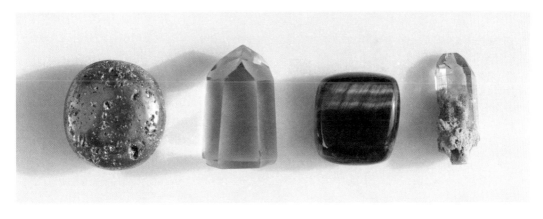

From left to right: pyrite, citrine, tiger's eye and topaz.

Tiger's Eye

A stone of confidence, bravery and willpower, tiger's eye is believed to carry the energies of the sun and earth combined. As a symbol of physical energy, this crystal awakens the solar plexus chakra and activates your inner fire, enhancing your resilience and your ability to act and succeed.

HOW TO USE THIS STONE
Carry tiger's eye when you need a boost of courage and motivation.

Topaz

Recognized as a stone of good luck, topaz can be used to attract prosperity and bounty. It is a powerful manifestation stone, working to amplify your intentions and activate the third energy centre. Symbolized by the sun god, Ra, in Egyptian philosophy, topaz balances the fire energy within our third chakra and enhances self-esteem and a positive mindset. Yellow and gold topaz are best suited here, while blue topaz activates the throat chakra, promoting self-expression and open communication (see also page 128).

HOW TO USE THIS STONE
Place it over the solar plexus chakra during meditation, and imagine its bright warming light activating this energy centre.

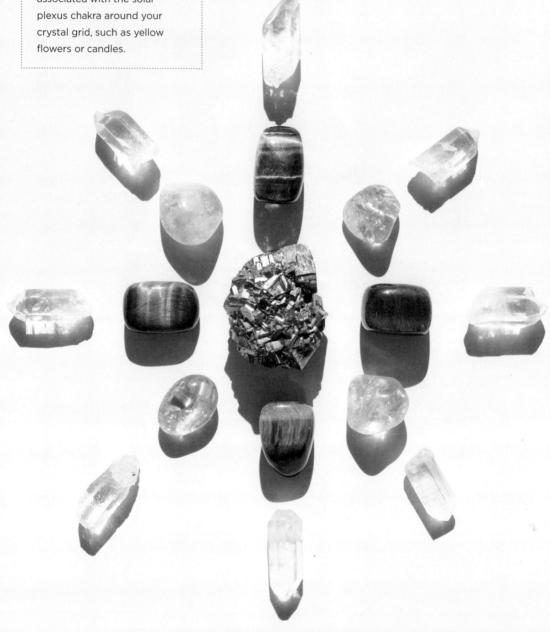

ENHANCE YOUR CHAKRA WORK: Arrange other elements associated with the solar plexus chakra around your crystal grid, such as yellow flowers or candles.

Crystal Grid for Prosperity

Use the empowering crystals in this crystal grid to strengthen your solar plexus chakra, boost your resilience and amplify energies of plenty and bounty. It is also effective for clearing negative energy from your space.

YOU WILL NEED

- A clean flat surface
- Energy cleansing toolkit (see page 50)
- 1 pyrite
- 4 tiger's eye
- 4 citrine (or smaller pyrite)
- 8 clear quartz

METHOD

1   Decide on a flat surface to keep your grid; this should be on a table or shelf that you can revisit, but which won't be in the way of your everyday life.
2   Cleanse the crystals and the space, following the instructions on page 50.
3   Set your intention for the grid, giving the crystals a specific purpose – for example, 'Abundance and success flow easily to me' or 'I am attracting wealth and success every day'.
4   Begin creating your grid, starting with the main centre crystal; in this case, pyrite.
5   Add the four tiger's eye crystals, placing one on each side of the pyrite.
6   Place your four citrine stones (or smaller pyrite) in between the tiger's eye crystals.
7   Now place each clear quartz crystal around the outside of the other stones to form a symmetrical pattern. Although it is not typically associated with the solar plexus chakra, clear quartz acts as an energy amplifier for the other stones.
8   Complete the process by focusing your energy on your intention for a minute or two. Visualize yourself feeling abundant, successful and full of gratitude.
9   Leave your grid in place for as long as you like, remembering to cleanse it occasionally and refocus your intention.

Bath for Alleviating Mental Fatigue

This empowering self-care ritual is designed to balance the solar plexus chakra. This bath is particularly beneficial if you are feeling drained or your emotions are out of balance.

YOU WILL NEED

- Energy cleansing toolkit (see page 50)
- Solar plexus chakra crystals (see page 94); note that pyrite should not be immersed in water due to its high iron content
- Sea salt or Epsom salts
- Solar plexus chakra flowers (see page 29)
- Lemon, ginger or chamomile tea
- Yellow beeswax or soy candles
- Calming music

METHOD

1　Cleanse the bathroom, following the instructions on page 50.
2　Run the bath, slowly adding in your healing crystals, bath salts and flowers. Add the herbal tea directly to your bath water, or save it to sip while you are bathing. Light your candles and play calming music to create a peaceful atmosphere.
3　Once you are comfortably in the bath, focus on your breathing. Close your eyes and visualize your solar plexus chakra as a bright spinning wheel of energy.
4　Let go of any tension in your body as you begin to feel centred. Choose an affirmation or intention relating to your third chakra – for example, 'I am full of joy and inner strength' – to meditate on as you attract new positive energy into your life.
5　Extinguish the candles safely.
6　Enjoy feeling rejuvenated, energized and present as you continue your day or evening.

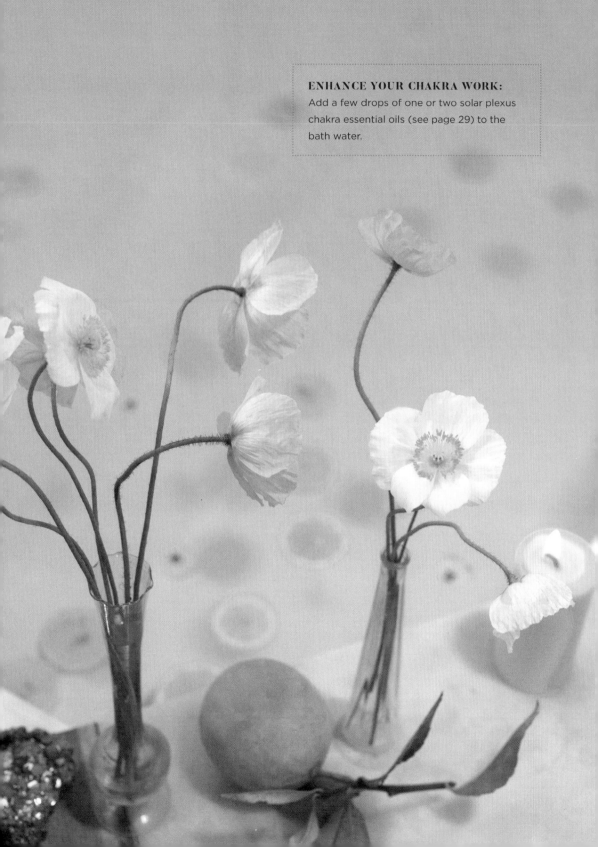

ENHANCE YOUR CHAKRA WORK:
Add a few drops of one or two solar plexus chakra essential oils (see page 29) to the bath water.

Ritual for Abundance

Try this ritual when you need to alleviate feelings of self-doubt and develop the confidence to achieve your goals.

YOU WILL NEED

- Energy cleansing toolkit (see page 50)
- Pen and paper
- One or more crystals corresponding to the solar plexus chakra (see page 94)
- Heatproof bowl
- Matches or lighter

METHOD

1 Find a quiet, comfortable place where you can meditate with no distractions. Cleanse the space, following the instructions on page 50.
2 Sit comfortably and take a few deep breaths to focus your energy. Think about what you would like to release to help you attract new energies of abundance; this could include negative habits that may be holding you back or unhelpful thought patterns.
3 Write down what you would like to release and add an intention, such as 'I am working towards my goals every day'.
4 Spend a couple of minutes meditating on your intentions while holding your crystal.
5 Focus on your solar plexus chakra and visualize a glowing yellow light expanding with each inhale. As you exhale, release any insecurity or doubt you may be holding on to. This will help strengthen your solar plexus chakra and develop greater confidence in yourself.
6 To complete the process, place the piece of paper in the heatproof bowl and burn it, along with all you intend to release. Ensure the flames are fully extinguished when you are finished.

Solar Plexus Chakra Journaling

This seven-day exercise will help you determine the health of your solar plexus chakra, while promoting a clearer understanding of your personal identity, confidence and sense of purpose. Answer one of the journal prompts below each day for a week, honouring any emotions and past experiences that come up during the process.

YOU WILL NEED

- Pen and journal

METHOD

1   Begin the exercise by sitting quietly for a few minutes, focusing on your breathing to centre your energy.
2   Pick one of the following questions and answer honestly, noticing the effect it has on you:
    - Would you consider yourself a confident person, and what does self-confidence mean to you?
    - How important are your values and self-worth: are you able to set boundaries and stick to them?
    - Do you feel empowered to pursue your goals towards success?
    - Are you comfortable following your own path or do you often feel unsure of your purpose?
    - Do you feel motivated in your life or do you lack the determination to move forward?
    - Do you crave validation from others or are you confident in your own individuality?
    - How can you cultivate a deeper sense of self-acceptance and confidence?
3   Write your responses in your journal, working through any thoughts or emotions that arise.
4   Sit for a moment and meditate on an intention to support your solar plexus chakra – for example, 'I am confident and powerful'.

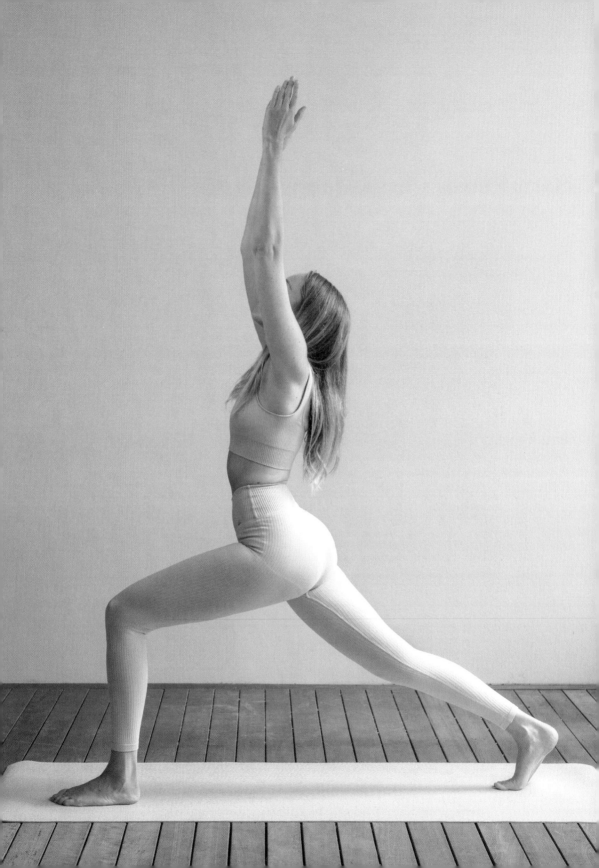

ENHANCE YOUR CHAKRA WORK:
Before you do this yoga pose, apply the
Essential Oil Blend for Self-confidence (see
page 90) to your wrists or over your solar
plexus chakra.

Yoga for Self-esteem

Associated with fire energy, the Warrior Pose (*Virabhadrasana* I) promotes
confidence and courage. Try this pose to draw upon your inner power when
you feel low in self-esteem.

YOU WILL NEED
- Comfortable, non-restrictive clothing
- Yoga mat

METHOD
1 Begin in a standing position with your hands at your heart centre.
2 As you exhale, step your left foot forward about 1.2m (4ft) into a lunge
   position, with your toes pointing forward and your right leg straight
   behind you.
3 Turn your right heel so that it is facing out towards your right, at about
   45 degrees. Alternatively, keep it facing forward if you find this more
   comfortable.
4 Keeping your shoulders down and facing forward, raise your arms straight
   above your head, with the palms facing in, and reach actively through
   your fingers.
5 Keeping your hips facing forward toward the front of the mat and your
   right heel grounded firmly on the floor, arch your upper torso slightly.
6 Lift your chin and look towards your hands. Hold this pose and spend 3–5
   breaths or longer here, focusing your energy into your solar plexus chakra.
7 Return to a standing position.
8 Repeat on the right side.

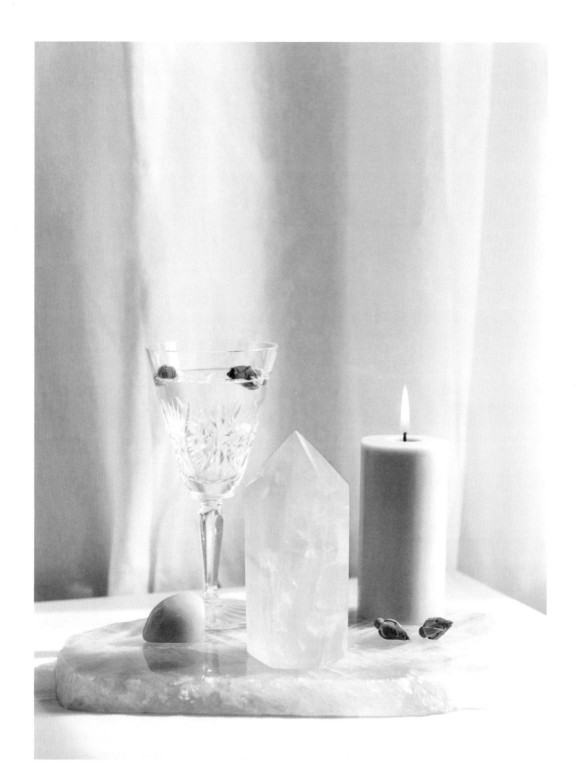

HEART CHAKRA

LOVE AND CONNECTION

Tea for Love

The centre of our love and connectedness to all things, the heart chakra promotes kindness, forgiveness, compassion and emotional healing. Use this beautiful infusion of hawthorn and rosehip when going through a difficult phase in a relationship to nurture your connection through openness, love and compassion.

YOU WILL NEED (INGREDIENTS PER CUP)

- 1 teaspoon dried hawthorn berries
- 1 teaspoon dried rosehips
- Teapot
- 400ml (13½fl oz) boiling water
- Cup
- Sweetener of your choice (optional)

METHOD

1   Put the hawthorn berries and rosehips into the teapot and pour over the boiling water.
2   Cover and leave the ingredients to steep for 5–10 minutes.
3   Pour the tea into the cup and add some sweetener, if desired.
4   Find somewhere peaceful to sit. While you drink the tea, focus on the intention of bringing love and open-heartedness.

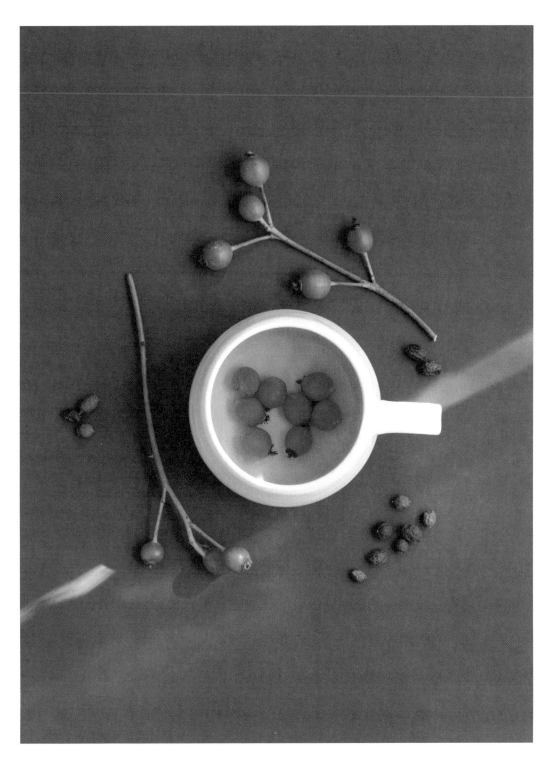

Essential Oil Blend for Self-love

Practising self-love is an important aspect of healing your heart chakra. Using essential oils that carry heart-opening and nurturing qualities is an effective way to restore this energy centre. Try this essential oil blend to develop greater self-love, forgiveness and acceptance for all parts of yourself, while also promoting emotional resilience and stress relief.

YOU WILL NEED

- 4 drops geranium essential oil
- 12 drops rose essential oil
- 4 drops hyssop essential oil
- 10-ml (⅓-fl oz) glass rollerball bottle
- Small funnel or dropper
- Carrier oil, such as almond, rosehip, argan or fractionated coconut oil
- Blank label
- Pen

METHOD

1. Add the essential oils to the rollerball bottle.
2. Using a small funnel or dropper, top up the bottle with the carrier oil.
3. Insert the rollerball, close the lid and swirl to combine.
4. Write a label and stick it to the bottle.
5. To use the blend, roll a small amount on the inside of your wrists in a circular motion, or apply directly to the heart chakra whenever you are in need of some self-love. You can also apply it before the Meditation for Emotional Support (see page 109) to enhance the practice.

ENHANCE YOUR CHAKRA WORK:
Hold a heart chakra crystal (see page 110)
in your hands during the meditation.

Meditation for Emotional Support

Designed to balance and energize the heart chakra, this restorative
meditation will help you feel open, connected and emotionally supported.
Try it when you need a renewed sense of strength, stability and harmony.

YOU WILL NEED

- Oil burner or diffuser
- Matches or lighter
- One or more heart chakra essential oils (see page 33)

METHOD

1 Find a quiet, comfortable place where you can meditate with no
distractions. Light the oil burner or diffuser and add the essential oils.

2 Sit in a comfortable position, with your spine straight and your shoulders
relaxed. Close your eyes and take a few deep breaths, allowing your mind
and body to relax completely. Feel the tension release from your face,
jaw, neck and shoulders right down to your toes.

3 Now bring your focus to your heart chakra, taking note of any feelings
that arise. Do you feel loved? Do you feel open and compassionate
towards yourself and others? Focus on feeling present in your body. Don't
worry if your mind wanders; just gently bring your attention back to
your breathing.

4 Visualize a green or pink light where your heart chakra resides. Imagine
this glowing ball of light growing brighter with each inhale.

5 As you exhale, release any hurt or mistrust you may be holding on to and
welcome in new forgiving, nurturing energy. Feel the aroma of essential
oils fill every cell in your body.

6 When you are ready to open your eyes, take a few deep breaths and
experience a sense of open-heartedness and healing, before bringing
awareness back to your surroundings.

7 Turn off the burner or diffuser.

Stones for Balancing the Heart Chakra

The heart chakra is the centre of love, compassion and healing. Its energy can be supported by stones that carry nurturing qualities, which can bring this chakra into balance. Use these crystals to help you work through unresolved emotions and bring loving energy into your life.

Rose Quartz

Recognized as the stone of unconditional love and compassion, rose quartz is a powerful crystal for activating the heart chakra. It is helpful for attracting new attachments, cultivating self-love and supporting current relationships. Opening the heart on all levels, it brings a clearer understanding of love and emotional healing.

HOW TO USE THIS STONE
Wear rose quartz in a necklace over the heart chakra to encourage self-love and acceptance.

Green Aventurine

Associated with the heart chakra, green aventurine encourages love, healing and forgiveness, while facilitating the release of unhealthy attachments. It carries a deeply nourishing energy that heals the fourth energy centre, bringing inner peace and acceptance.

HOW TO USE THIS STONE
Carry green aventurine to attract positivity into your life and to encourage personal growth.

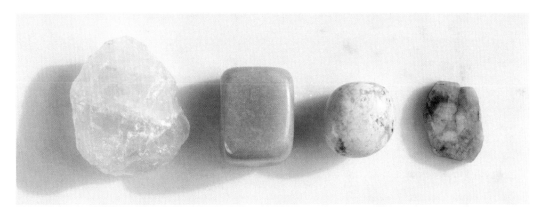

From left to right: rose quartz, green aventurine, rhodochrosite and emerald.

Rhodochrosite

With its beautiful pink hue and peaceful energy, rhodochrosite is an ideal crystal for self-love and emotional healing. Associated with the heart chakra, this stone promotes affection and forgiveness, while encouraging deeper commitment and unconditional love.

HOW TO USE THIS STONE
Use rhodochrosite during meditation to activate the heart chakra and bring in new energies of affection, compassion and healing.

Emerald

Recognized as the 'stone of successful love', emerald activates the heart chakra and teaches generosity, commitment and compassion. This crystal brings fresh energy to a relationship, boosting romantic partnerships and healing the connection with yourself.

HOW TO USE THIS STONE
Place emerald over the heart chakra during meditation to facilitate emotional healing and instil patience.

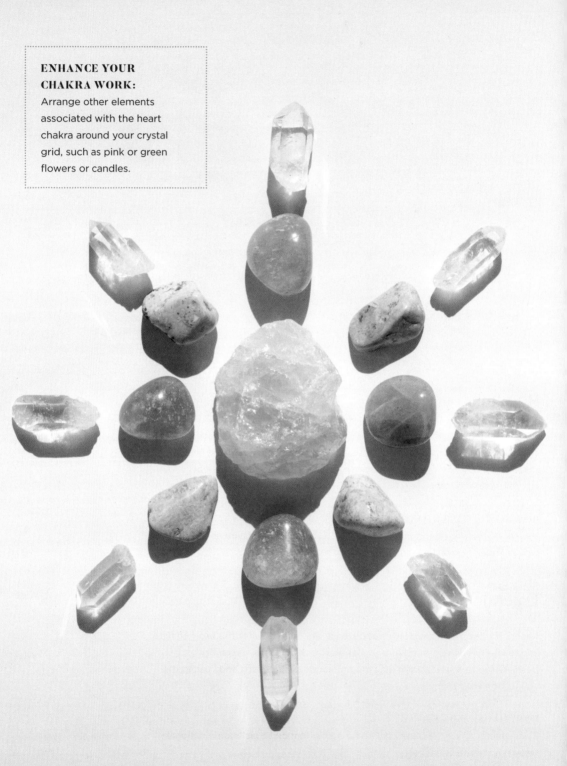

**ENHANCE YOUR
CHAKRA WORK:**
Arrange other elements
associated with the heart
chakra around your crystal
grid, such as pink or green
flowers or candles.

Crystal Grid for Connection

This crystal grid can be used to help focus your intention on healing unprocessed emotions in order to strengthen the heart chakra. The stones used in this grid carry nurturing energies of love and connection, and are helpful for balancing this energy centre. Try this exercise if you feel emotionally disconnected or closed off from others.

YOU WILL NEED

- A clean flat surface
- Energy cleansing toolkit (see page 50)
- 1 rose quartz
- 4 green aventurine
- 4 rhodochrosite (or smaller rose quartz)
- 8 clear quartz

METHOD

1   Decide on a flat surface to keep your grid; this should be on a table or shelf that you can revisit, but which won't be in the way of your everyday life.

2   Cleanse the crystals and the space, following the instructions on page 50.

3   Set your intention for the grid, giving the crystals a specific purpose – for example, 'Love and connection flow easily to me' or 'I am open to love'.

4   Begin creating your grid, starting with the main centre crystal; in this case, rose quartz.

5   Add the four green aventurine stones, placing one on each side of the rose quartz.

6   Place your four rhodochrosite crystals (or smaller rose quartz) in between the green aventurine.

7   Now place each clear quartz crystal around the outside of the other stones to form a symmetrical pattern. Although it is not typically associated with the heart chakra, clear quartz acts as an energy amplifier for the other stones.

8   Complete the process by focusing your energy on your intention for a minute or two. Visualize yourself feeling loved, open-hearted and connected to the world around you.

9   Leave your grid in place for as long as you like, remembering to cleanse it occasionally and to refocus your intention.

ENHANCE YOUR CHAKRA WORK:
Add a few drops of one or two heart
chakra essential oils (see page 33) to
the bath water.

Bath for Attracting Loving Energy

Try this nurturing bathing ritual when you are in need of a greater sense of
love and connection, or when struggling to process your emotions.

YOU WILL NEED
- Energy cleansing toolkit (see page 50)
- Heart chakra crystals (see page 110)
- Sea salt or Epsom salts
- Heart chakra flowers (see page 33)
- Rosehip or hawthorn berry tea
- Pink or green beeswax or soy candles
- Calming music

METHOD
1   Cleanse the bathroom, following the instructions on page 50.
2   Run the bath, slowly adding in your healing crystals, bath salts and
    flowers. Add the herbal tea directly to your bath water, or save it to sip
    while you are bathing. Light your candles and play calming music to
    create a peaceful atmosphere.
3   Once you are comfortably in the bath, focus on your breathing. Close
    your eyes and visualize your heart chakra as a bright spinning wheel
    of energy.
4   Let go of any tension in your body as you begin to feel centred. Choose
    an affirmation or intention relating to your fourth chakra – for example,
    'I have an open heart' or 'I choose love always' – to meditate on as you
    attract new positive and loving energy into your life.
5   Extinguish the candles safely.
6   Enjoy feeling a deeper sense of love, trust and connection as you
    continue your day or evening.

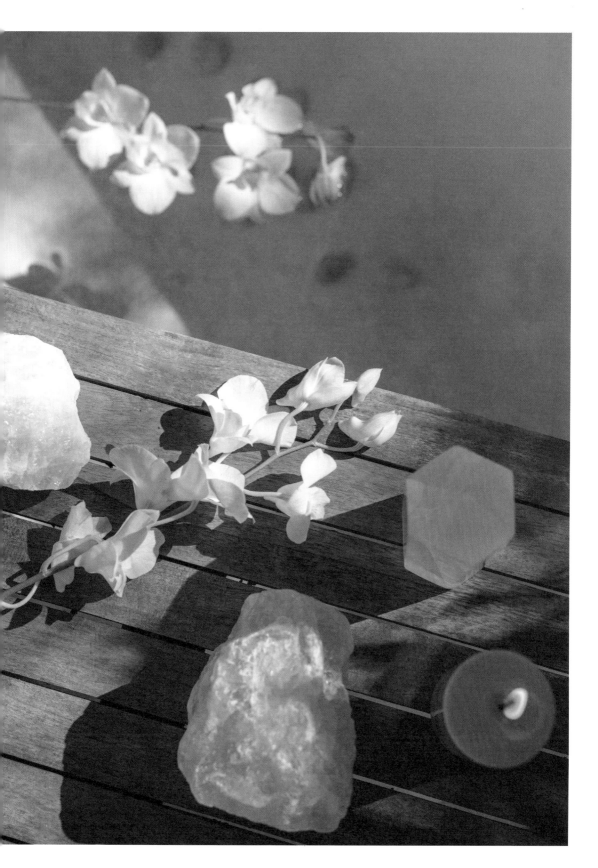

Ritual for Heart Healing

The heart chakra is responsible for our relationships. Try this ritual to release unhealthy attachments and to heal yourself of past negative experiences.

YOU WILL NEED

- Energy cleansing toolkit (see page 50)
- Pen and paper
- One or more crystals corresponding to the heart chakra (see page 110)
- Heatproof bowl
- Matches or lighter

METHOD

1 Find a quiet, comfortable place where you can meditate with no distractions. Cleanse the space, following the instructions on page 50.
2 Sit comfortably and take a few deep breaths to focus your energy. Think about what you would like to release to help you attract new energy into your life; this could include unhealthy attachments or unhelpful thought patterns.
3 Write down what you would like to let go of and add an intention, such as 'I release all unhealthy relationships from my past' or 'I attract only loving connections into my life'.
4 Spend a couple of minutes meditating on your intentions while holding your crystal.
5 Focus on your heart chakra and visualize a glowing pink or green light, expanding with each inhale. As you exhale, release any emotional pain or attachments you may be holding on to. This will help you make room for new energies of love and connection.
6 To complete the process, place the piece of paper in the heatproof bowl and burn it, along with all you intend to release. Ensure the flames are fully extinguished when you are finished.

Heart Chakra Journaling

This seven-day exercise will help you determine the health of your heart chakra, while allowing you to release unprocessed emotions relating to your openness to express love, forgiveness and empathy. Answer one of the journal prompts below each day for a week, honouring any emotions and past experiences that come up in the process.

YOU WILL NEED

- Pen and journal

METHOD

1 Begin the exercise by sitting quietly for a few minutes, focusing on your breathing to centre your energy.
2 Pick one of the following questions and answer honestly, noticing the effect it has on you:
   - Are you able to openly express love and compassion?
   - What does self-love mean to you?
   - Are you able to forgive others or are you prone to holding on to past hurt?
   - Do you engage in negative self-talk or unhelpful thought patterns or do you accept yourself unconditionally?
   - Do you find it difficult to open yourself up and trust others?
   - Are you able to set clear boundaries in relationships?
   - How are you able to live more consciously from a place of love and compassion?
3 Write your responses in your journal, working through any thoughts or emotions that arise.
4 Sit for a moment and meditate on an intention to support your heart chakra – for example, 'I am open to love and connection'.

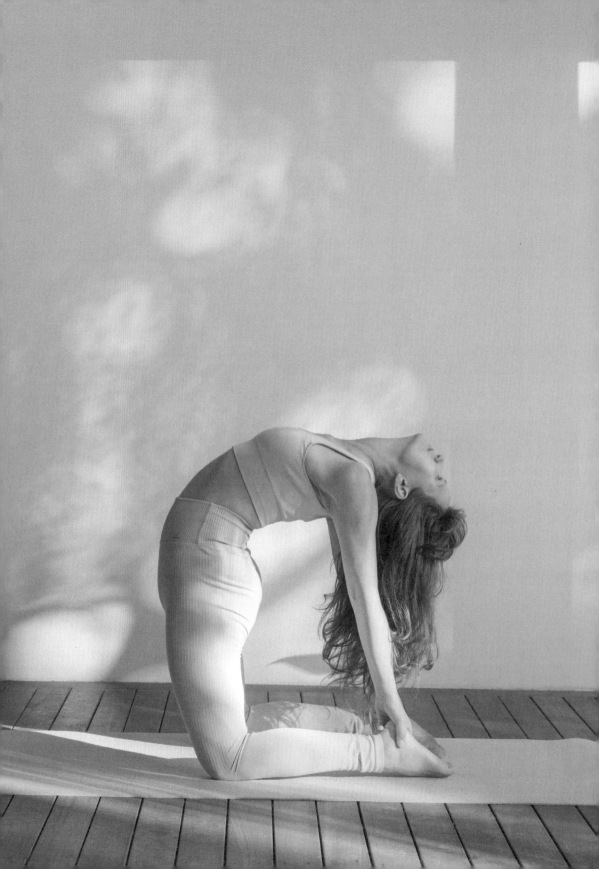

ENHANCE YOUR CHAKRA WORK:
Before you do this yoga pose, apply the
Essential Oil Blend for Self-love (see page
108) to your wrists or over your heart chakra.

Yoga for an Open Heart

Known as a heart-opening position, the Camel Pose (*Ustrasana*) stretches
the front of the body and opens the chest. Try this pose when you feel
emotionally closed off from others. It will create openness in your heart
centre, allowing energy to flow freely while strengthening the link between
your higher and lower chakras.

YOU WILL NEED

- Comfortable, non-restrictive clothing
- Yoga mat

METHOD

1 Kneel with your shoulders over your hips, creating a straight line to
   your knees.
2 Rest your palms on your lower back, pressing your hips forward, then
   begin leaning back, opening your heart space.
3 Place your hands on the floor behind you or hold your heels for balance.
4 As you inhale, bring one hand up to your heart chakra.
5 Spend 3–5 breaths or longer here, focusing your energy into this chakra.
6 To complete the pose, activate your core and slowly move back up into a
   kneeling position.

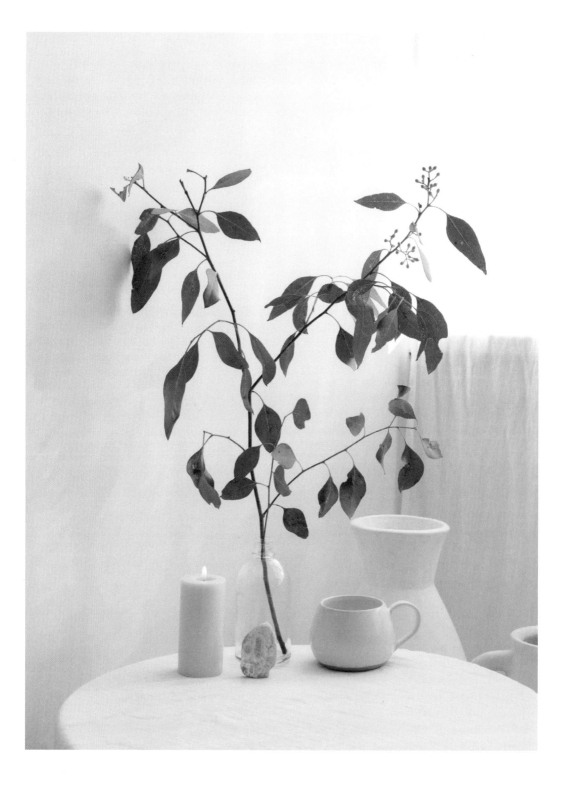

THROAT CHAKRA

COMMUNICATION AND EXPRESSION

Tea for Truth

The throat chakra is associated with communication, self-expression and honesty. This powerful blend of peppermint and sage will activate the throat chakra and help you to master the power of truthful communication. Try drinking this tea whenever you feel restricted in the way you speak.

YOU WILL NEED (INGREDIENTS PER CUP)
- 1 teaspoon dried peppermint leaves
- 1 teaspoon dried sage leaves
- Teapot
- 400ml (13½fl oz) boiling water
- Cup
- Sweetener of your choice (optional)

METHOD
1 Put the herbs into the teapot and pour over the boiling water.
2 Cover and leave the ingredients to steep for 5–10 minutes.
3 Pour the tea into the cup and add some sweetener, if desired.
4 Find somewhere peaceful to sit. While you drink the tea, focus on the intention of bringing truth and open communication.

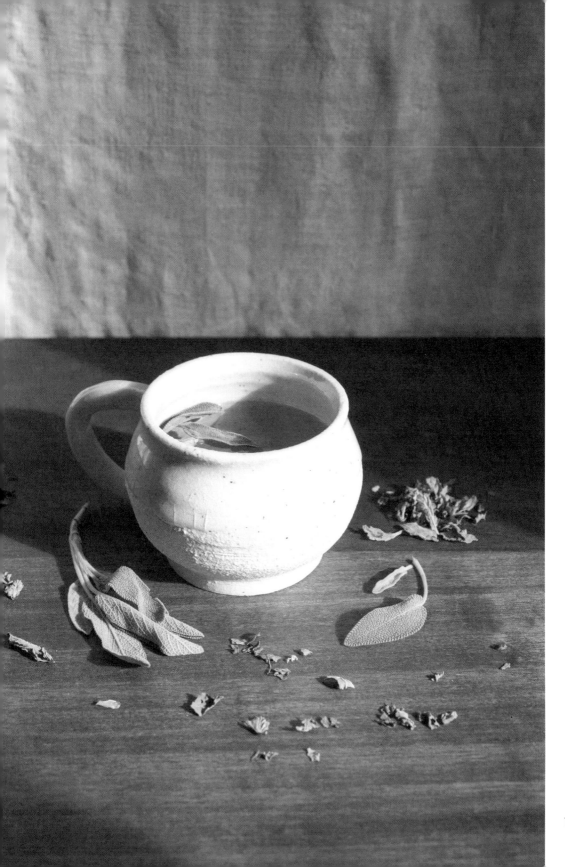

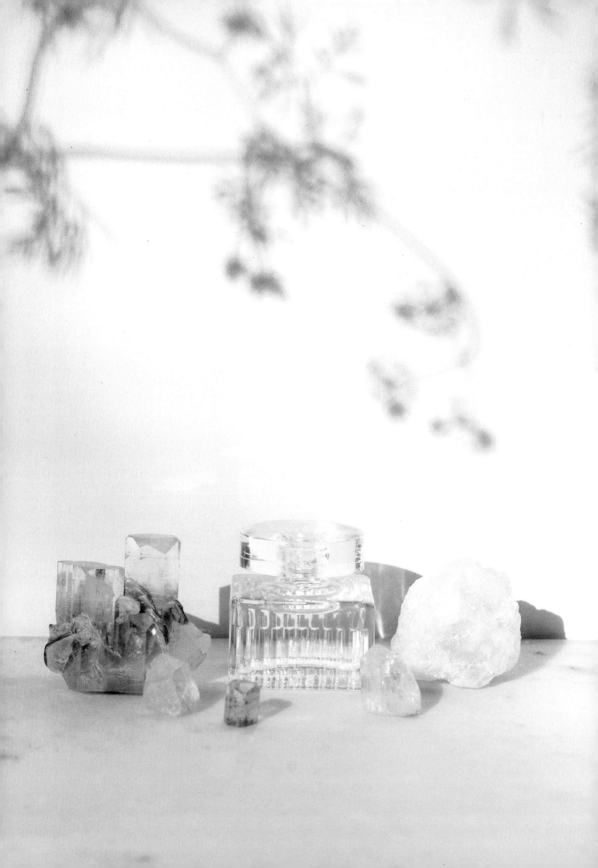

ENHANCE YOUR CHAKRA WORK:
Add a peppermint leaf or a small throat chakra crystal (see page 128) to the bottle.

Essential Oil Blend for Open Communication

When this energy centre is closed, you may have difficulty explaining your thoughts and opinions in a constructive way, or find it hard to share your feelings without fear of judgement. Use this essential oil blend to inspire open and mindful communication.

YOU WILL NEED

- 4 drops eucalyptus essential oil
- 12 drops peppermint essential oil
- 4 drops tea tree essential oil
- 10-ml (⅓-fl oz) glass rollerball bottle
- Small funnel or dropper
- Carrier oil, such as almond, rosehip, argan or fractionated coconut oil
- Blank label
- Pen

METHOD

1 Add the essential oils to the rollerball bottle.
2 Using a small funnel or dropper, top up the bottle with the carrier oil.
3 Insert the rollerball, close the lid and swirl to combine.
4 Write a label and stick it to the bottle.
5 To use the blend, roll a small amount on the inside of your wrists in a circular motion, or apply directly to the throat chakra whenever you wish to strengthen your communication skills. You can also apply before the Meditation for Self-doubt (see page 126) to enhance the practice.

ENHANCE YOUR CHAKRA WORK:
Hold a throat chakra crystal (see page 128) in your hands during the meditation.

Meditation for Self-doubt

This meditation is designed to activate the throat chakra. It will also encourage honest self-expression by alleviating anxiety and self-doubt.

YOU WILL NEED

- Oil burner or diffuser
- Matches or lighter
- One or more throat chakra essential oils (see page 37)

METHOD

1 Find a quiet, comfortable place where you can meditate with no distractions. Light the oil burner or diffuser and add the essential oils.
2 Sit in a comfortable position, with your spine straight and your shoulders relaxed. Close your eyes and take a few deep breaths, allowing your mind and body to relax completely. Feel the tension release from your face, jaw, neck and shoulders right down to your toes.
3 Now bring your focus to your throat chakra, taking note of any feelings that arise. Do you feel open to express yourself? Are you free to share your inner truth? Focus on feeling present in your body. Don't worry if your mind wanders; just gently bring your attention back to your breathing.
4 Visualize a blue light where your throat chakra resides. Imagine this glowing ball of light growing brighter with each inhale.
5 As you exhale, release any insecurities or concerns about communication, and feel safe to express yourself openly. Feel the aroma of the essential oils fill every cell in your body.
6 When you are ready to open your eyes, take a few deep breaths and experience a sense of openness and understanding, before bringing awareness back to your surroundings.
7 Turn off the burner or diffuser.

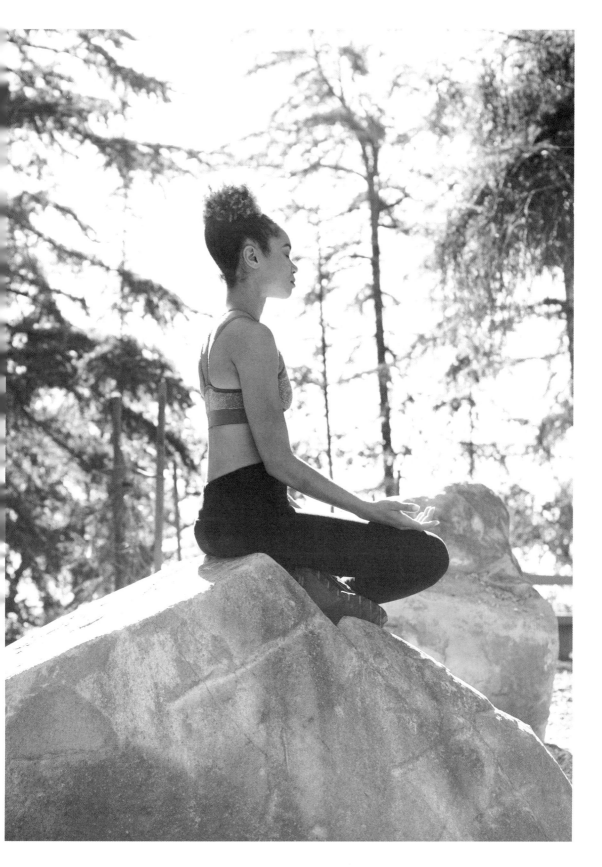

Stones for Balancing the Throat Chakra

The throat chakra teaches the power of affirmation and is responsible for our communication and authentic truth. This energy centre can be supported by crystals and gemstones that have healing properties related to self-expression. Use these stones to help heal your fifth energy centre and welcome in new energies of open discourse and understanding.

Larimar

Larimar supports the throat chakra by alleviating patterns of fear, panic and anxiety around communication. This stone's stabilizing energy makes it an effective tool for calming nervous energy. Larimar works to remove energy blockages from the fifth chakra to encourage truthful self-expression so that you are able to communicate openly without fear.

HOW TO USE THIS STONE
Wear larimar in a necklace to calm nervous energy and dissolve feelings of fear when expressing yourself openly.

Amazonite

Amazonite is a stone of empowerment and personal development, making it an effective tool for enhancing the energy of the throat chakra. Known as a 'stone of truth', it will bring honest and open dialogue to all aspects of your life. With its calming energy, amazonite also brings focus, so that you can learn to express yourself in a clear, concise manner.

HOW TO USE THIS STONE
Use amazonite in a crystal grid to alleviate the fear of judgement and worry surrounding communication and self-expression.

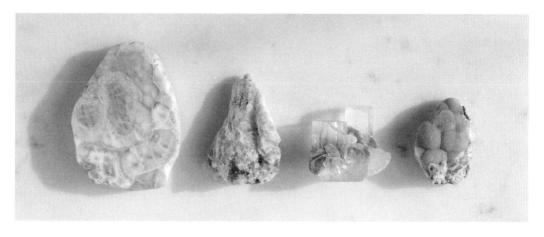
From left to right: larimar, amazonite, aquamarine and hemimorphite.

Aquamarine

A powerful throat chakra stone, aquamarine enhances all types of communication. It brings clarity to the mind so that you can express yourself in a thoughtful way. If you find yourself speaking without thinking, aquamarine can help centre your energy so that you stay present and speak with intention.

HOW TO USE THIS STONE
Use aquamarine during meditation to activate the fifth energy centre and connect to your deepest truth. This stone will enable you to share your feelings without fear of criticism.

Hemimorphite

This is an excellent stone for maintaining healthy relationships, as it encourages open dialogue, understanding and empathy between two people. Its gentle energy teaches patience and allows unstable relationships to heal. Linked to the fifth energy centre, this crystal promotes truthfulness.

HOW TO USE THIS STONE
Carry hemimorphite with you when you find yourself struggling to convey your needs effectively in a relationship.

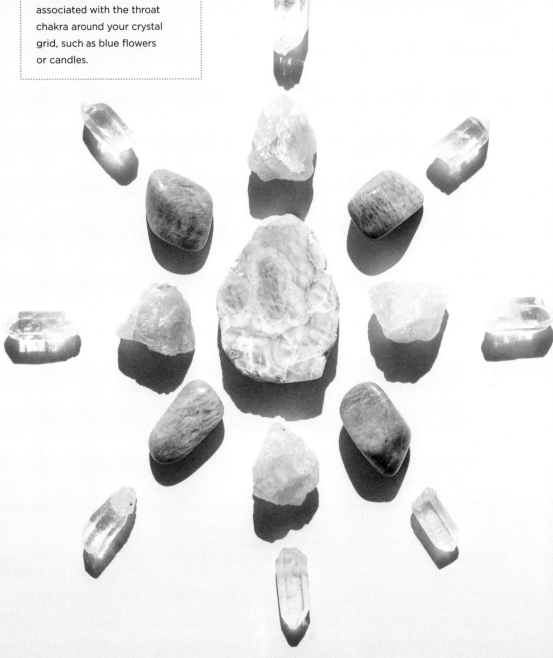

**ENHANCE YOUR
CHAKRA WORK:**
Arrange other elements
associated with the throat
chakra around your crystal
grid, such as blue flowers
or candles.

Crystal Grid for Authentic Truth

The stones in this crystal grid carry purifying energies associated with truth, understanding and integrity and offer a powerful combination for strengthening the throat chakra. Use this exercise if you are struggling to feel heard or are looking to calm your emotions in order to speak freely and concisely.

YOU WILL NEED

- A clean flat surface
- Energy cleansing toolkit (see page 50)
- 1 larimar
- 4 aquamarine
- 4 amazonite (or smaller larimar)
- 8 clear quartz

METHOD

1 Decide on a flat surface to keep your grid; this should be on a table or shelf that you can revisit, but which won't be in the way of your everyday life.

2 Cleanse the crystals and the space, following the instructions on page 50.

3 Set your intention for the grid, giving the crystals a specific purpose – for example, 'I speak with confidence' or 'I communicate with intention.'

4 Begin creating your grid, starting with the main centre crystal; in this case, larimar.

5 Add the four aquamarine stones, placing one on each side of the larimar.

6 Place your four amazonite crystals (or smaller larimar) in between the aquamarine.

7 Now place each clear quartz crystal around the outside of the other stones to form a symmetrical pattern. Although it is not typically associated with the throat chakra, clear quartz acts as an energy amplifier for the other stones.

8 Complete the process by focusing your energy on your intention for a minute or two. Visualize yourself feeling confident to express yourself authentically without fear.

9 Leave your grid in place for as long as you like, remembering to cleanse it occasionally and to refocus your intention.

ENHANCE YOUR CHAKRA WORK:
Add a few drops of one or two throat chakra
essential oils (see page 37) to the bath water.

Bath for Self-assurance

Find comfort in this ritual when you feel fearful or anxious about speaking
openly and confidently, or if you find yourself in a habit of negative self-talk.

YOU WILL NEED

- Energy cleansing toolkit (see page 50)
- Throat chakra crystals (see page 128)
- Sea salt or Epsom salts
- Throat chakra flowers (see page 37)
- Sage or peppermint tea
- Blue beeswax or soy candles
- Calming music

METHOD

1 Cleanse the bathroom, following the instructions on page 50.
2 Run the bath, slowly adding in your healing crystals, bath salts and
   flowers. Add the herbal tea directly to your bath water, or save it to sip
   while you are bathing. Light your candles and play calming music to
   create a peaceful atmosphere.
3 Once you are comfortably in the bath, focus on your breathing. Close
   your eyes and visualize your throat chakra as a bright spinning wheel
   of energy.
4 Let go of any tension in your body as you begin to feel centred. Choose
   an affirmation or intention relating to your fifth chakra – for example,
   'I speak with confidence' or 'I live and speak my authentic truth' – to
   meditate on as you attract new positive and clear energy into your life.
5 Extinguish the candles safely.
6 Enjoy feeling a deeper connection to your inner truth and powerful
   self-expression.

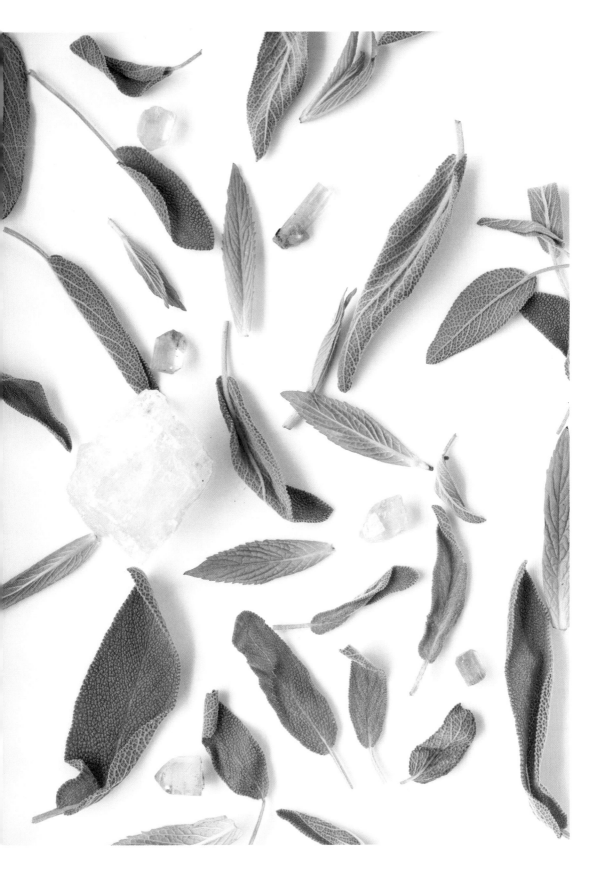

Ritual for Truthful Expression

Try this ritual to release old, problematic ways of communicating, so that you can feel confident to convey your thoughts.

YOU WILL NEED

- Energy cleansing toolkit (see page 50)
- Pen and paper
- One or more crystals corresponding to the throat chakra (see page 128)
- Heatproof bowl
- Matches or lighter

METHOD

1   Find a quiet, comfortable place where you can meditate with no distractions. Cleanse the space, following the instructions on page 50.

2   Sit comfortably and take a few deep breaths to focus your energy. Think about what you would like to release, including limiting beliefs from your past, patterns you need to unlearn or moments when you felt insecure or unable to express yourself.

3   Write down what you would like to overcome and add an intention, such as 'I speak from a place of confidence' or 'I choose to overcome my past unhelpful beliefs'.

4   Spend a couple of minutes meditating on your intentions while holding your crystal.

5   Focus on your throat chakra and visualize a glowing blue light expanding with each inhale. As you exhale, release any unhelpful beliefs relating to communication and expression. This will help make room for new opportunities and connections.

6   To complete the process, place the piece of paper in the heatproof bowl and burn it, along with all you intend to release. Ensure the flames are fully extinguished when you are finished.

Throat Chakra Journaling

This seven-day exercise will help you determine the health of your throat chakra, while promoting a clearer understanding of your authentic truth and open dialogue. Answer one of the journal prompts below each day for a week, honouring any emotions and past experiences that come up during the process.

YOU WILL NEED
- Pen and journal

METHOD
1   Begin the exercise by sitting quietly for a few minutes, focusing on your breathing to centre your energy.
2   Pick one of the following questions and answer honestly, noticing the effect it has on you:
    - Are you able to communicate your thoughts clearly and confidently?
    - Do you speak your honest truth or do you find it difficult to express yourself?
    - Do you experience social anxiety and avoid situations where you may have to speak openly?
    - Do you have a healthy internal dialogue or do you often experience negative self-talk?
    - Did you grow up in an environment that was supportive of your self-expression or did you feel insecurity around honest communication?
    - Do you accept your true self or do you often hold back and make yourself smaller?
    - What can you do to gain more confidence around communicating openly and honestly?
3   Write your responses in your journal, working through any thoughts or emotions that arise.
4   Sit for a moment and meditate on an intention to support your throat chakra – for example, 'I speak truthfully and confidently'.

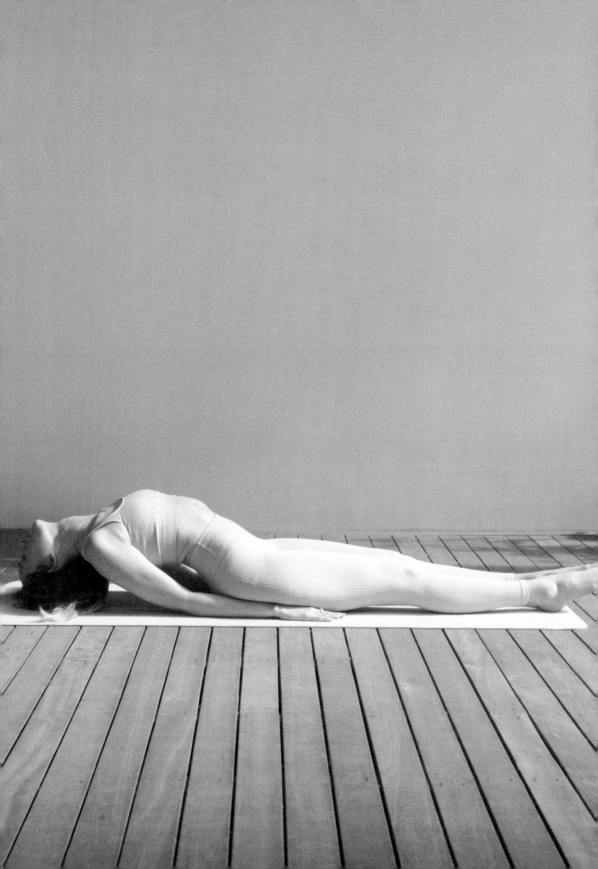

ENHANCE YOUR CHAKRA WORK:
Before you do this yoga pose, apply the
Essential Oil Blend for Open Communication
(see page 125) to your wrists or over your
throat chakra.

Yoga for Honesty

The Fish Pose (*Matsyasana*) releases tension in the neck and throat area
while strengthening and toning the upper back and shoulders. Try this
pose to open your fifth energy centre as a way to inspire honesty and trust
in relationships.

YOU WILL NEED

- Comfortable, non-restrictive clothing
- Yoga mat

METHOD

1   Start the position lying on your back, with your legs straight, your feet
    pointed and your body relaxed.
2   Slide your hands underneath your hips, so that your palms are flat on the
    floor and your elbows are pressed closely to your sides.
3   As you inhale, lift your chest, press your shoulder blades together and
    arch your back, making sure that you support your weight on your elbows
    and forearms.
4   Tilting your neck slowly, let the back of your head gently rest on the
    floor, keeping your chest lifted. You can also add a towel or bolster pillow
    behind your neck or back for extra support.
5   Press your thighs and legs to the floor, reaching out through your toes,
    and hold for 3–5 breaths or longer.
6   As you exhale, lower your back to the floor and straighten your neck to
    complete the exercise.

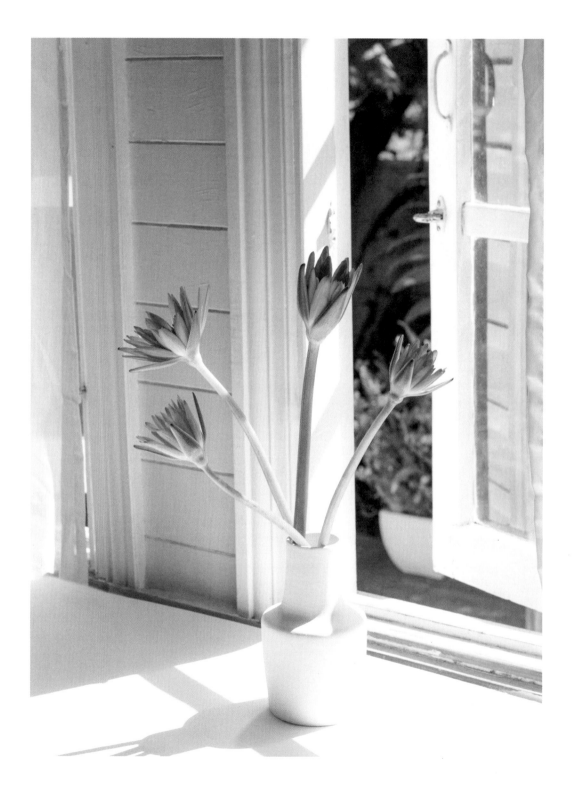

THIRD EYE
CHAKRA

KNOWLEDGE AND INTUITION

TRY THIS: For a tea to promote sleep and inspire dreams, replace the blue lotus flower and jasmine with 1 teaspoon dried eyebright and 1 teaspoon dried passionflower.

Tea for Insight

The sixth energy centre is responsible for our thoughts, dreams, insight and intuition. Try this floral infusion to gain greater spiritual connection and self-awareness while also releasing tension and anxiety.

YOU WILL NEED (INGREDIENTS PER CUP)

- 1 teaspoon dried blue lotus flowers
- 1 teaspoon dried jasmine flowers
- Teapot
- 400ml (13½fl oz) boiling water
- Cup
- Sweetener of your choice (optional)

METHOD

1 Put the flowers into the teapot and pour over the boiling water.
2 Cover and leave the ingredients to steep for 5–10 minutes.
3 Pour the tea into the cup and add some sweetener, if desired.
4 Find somewhere peaceful to sit. While you drink the tea, focus on the intention of strengthening your intuition and higher knowing.

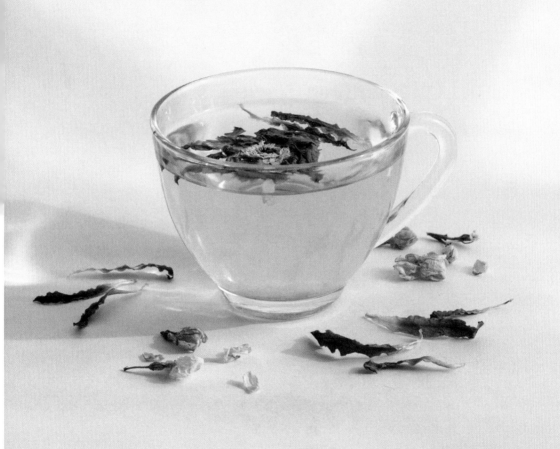

ENHANCE YOUR CHAKRA WORK:
Add a blue lotus petal or a small third eye
chakra crystal (see page 144) to the bottle.

Essential Oil Blend for Clarity

This energy centre is where our beliefs, values, thoughts and ideas are
developed. Use this essential oil blend to strengthen your sixth sense and
help you see things clearly. Apply before bed to experience vivid dreams.

YOU WILL NEED

- 2 drops rosemary essential oil
- 12 drops blue lotus essential oil
- 6 drops jasmine essential oil
- 10-ml (⅓-fl oz) glass rollerball bottle
- Small funnel or dropper
- Carrier oil such as almond, rosehip, argan or fractionated coconut
- Blank label
- Pen

METHOD

1   Add the essential oils to the rollerball bottle.
2   Using a small funnel or dropper, top up the bottle with the carrier oil.
3   Insert the rollerball, close the lid and swirl to combine.
4   Write a label and stick it to the bottle.
5   To use the blend, roll a small amount on the inside of your wrists in a
    circular motion, or apply directly to the third eye chakra to enhance
    mental clarity. You can also apply it before the Meditation for Perception
    (see page 143) to enhance the practice.

ENHANCE YOUR CHAKRA WORK:
Hold a third eye chakra crystal (see page 144) in your hands during the meditation.

Meditation for Perception

This powerful meditation is designed to strengthen your innate faith and ability to perceive subtle energy. Use it to enhance your psychic ability when seeking guidance with difficult decisions.

YOU WILL NEED

- Oil burner or diffuser
- Matches or lighter
- One or more third eye chakra essential oils (see page 41)

METHOD

1 Find a quiet, comfortable place where you can meditate with no distractions. Light the oil burner or diffuser and add the essential oils.

2 Sit in a comfortable position, with your spine straight and your shoulders relaxed. Close your eyes and take a few deep breaths, allowing your mind and body to relax completely. Feel the tension release from your face, jaw, neck and shoulders right down to your toes.

3 Now bring your focus to your third eye chakra, taking note of any feelings that arise. Do you feel intuitive and perceptive? Do you have a strong sense of spiritual awareness? Focus on feeling present in your body. Don't worry if your mind wanders; just gently bring your attention back to your breathing .

4 Visualize an indigo or purple light where your third eye chakra resides. Imagine this glowing ball of light growing brighter with each inhale.

5 As you exhale, release any limiting beliefs or stagnant energy relating to your intuition, and discover a new sense of perception and inner knowing. Feel the aroma of essential oils fill every cell in your body.

6 When you are ready to open your eyes, take a few deep breaths and experience a clearer sense of insight, before bringing your awareness back to your surroundings.

7 Turn off the burner or diffuser.

Stones for Balancing
the Third Eye Chakra

The third eye chakra enables us to connect with spirit guides, ignite our intuition and develop psychic abilities. This energy centre can be supported by crystals and gemstones that carry healing properties of insight and perception. Use these crystals to strengthen this chakra and calm the mind and to connect with your third eye energy.

Labradorite

Labradorite can help you harness the power of your third eye and is a powerful stone of personal transformation and new possibilities. Believed in various cultures to be a magic crystal, it carries protective, healing and spiritual expansion properties. Its energy eliminates negative energies and unhelpful thought patterns, enabling you to transform mentally and spiritually.

HOW TO USE THIS STONE
Carry labradorite with you to connect to its mystical energy and raise your vibration to a higher state of being.

Sodalite

Associated with the third eye chakra, sodalite strengthens intuition and promotes deeper knowledge and understanding. Its calm and stable energy allows for patience and reflection, helping to eliminate hesitation and confusion. Sodalite also promotes mental clarity and focus.

HOW TO USE THIS STONE
If you find it difficult to trust in your intuition, consider meditating with sodalite to strengthen your third eye chakra energy.

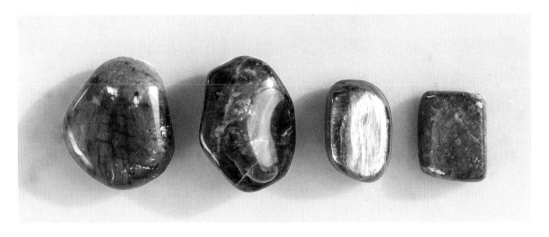

From left to right: labradorite, sodalite, blue kyanite and lapis lazuli.

Blue Kyanite

Blue kyanite carries a high spiritual vibration that can be used to facilitate the spiritual development and mental clarity associated with this chakra. Its energy can also be used to assist dream recall and lucid dreaming, helping to establish self-understanding, desires and present needs, as well as making contact with spirit guides.

HOW TO USE THIS STONE
Place kyanite under your pillow when you sleep to promote dream recall and enhance psychic abilities.

Lapis Lazuli

Recognized as a powerful amplifier of thought and intuition, lapis lazuli is strongly associated with the third eye chakra. Its energy encourages deep inner peace and enhances spiritual enlightenment. As a stone of knowledge and power, it can also be used to heighten intelligence.

HOW TO USE THIS STONE
Wear lapis lazuli to enhance intuition, wisdom and spiritual development.

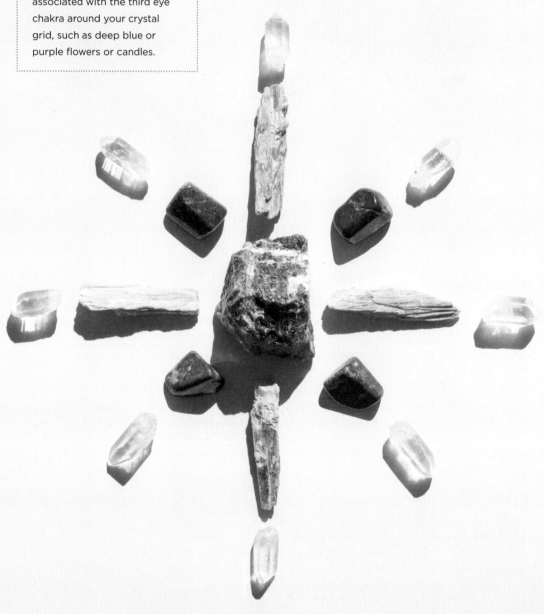

Crystal Grid for Inner Knowing

The crystals selected for this grid carry powerful third eye enhancing qualities that are known to heighten psychic ability. Try this exercise as a way to clear your mind and build trust in your inner knowing, particularly when seeking guidance and direction in life.

YOU WILL NEED

- A clean flat surface
- Energy cleansing toolkit (see page 50)
- 1 sodalite
- 4 blue kyanite
- 4 lapis lazuli (or smaller sodalite)
- 8 clear quartz

METHOD

1 Decide on a flat surface to keep your grid; this should be on a table or shelf that you can revisit, but which won't be in the way of your everyday life.

2 Cleanse the crystals and the space, following the instructions on page 50.

3 Set your intention for the grid, giving the crystals a specific purpose – for example, 'I am insightful and intuitive' or 'I am open to inner guidance'.

4 Begin creating your grid, starting with the main centre crystal; in this case, sodalite.

5 Add the four blue kyanite stones, placing one on each side of the sodalite.

6 Place your four lapis lazuli crystals (or sodalite) in between the kyanite.

7 Now place each clear quartz crystal around the outside of the other stones to form a symmetrical pattern. Although it is not typically associated with the throat chakra, clear quartz acts as an energy amplifier for the other stones.

8 Complete the process by focusing your energy on your intention for a minute or two. Visualize yourself feeling filled with inner knowing.

9 Leave your grid in place for as long as you like, remembering to cleanse it occasionally and to refocus your intention.

Bath for Calming the Mind

This relaxing self-care ritual is designed to quieten the mind and draw your focus inward. It will also activate the third eye chakra by means of elements connected to spiritual awareness, such as rosemary, lapis lazuli crystals and indigo or purple candles.

YOU WILL NEED

- Energy cleansing toolkit (see page 50)
- Third eye chakra crystals (see page 144); note that lapis lazuli, labradorite and kyanite should be placed around the bath and not immersed in water
- Sea salt or Epsom salts
- Third eye chakra flowers (see page 41)
- Blue lotus or jasmine tea
- Blue or purple beeswax or soy candles
- Calming music

METHOD

1 Cleanse the bathroom, following the instructions on page 50.
2 Run the bath, slowly adding in your healing crystals, bath salts and flowers. Add the herbal tea directly to your bath water, or save it to sip while you are bathing. Light your candles and play calming music to create a peaceful atmosphere.
3 Once you are comfortably in the bath, focus on your breathing. Close your eyes and visualize your third eye chakra as a bright spinning wheel of energy.
4 Let go of any tension in your body as you begin to feel centred. Choose an affirmation or intention relating to your sixth chakra - for example, 'I am insightful and intuitive' or 'I see and think clearly' - to meditate on as you attract powerful new energy.
5 Extinguish the candles safely.
6 Enjoy feeling a deeper connection to your inner knowing and insight.

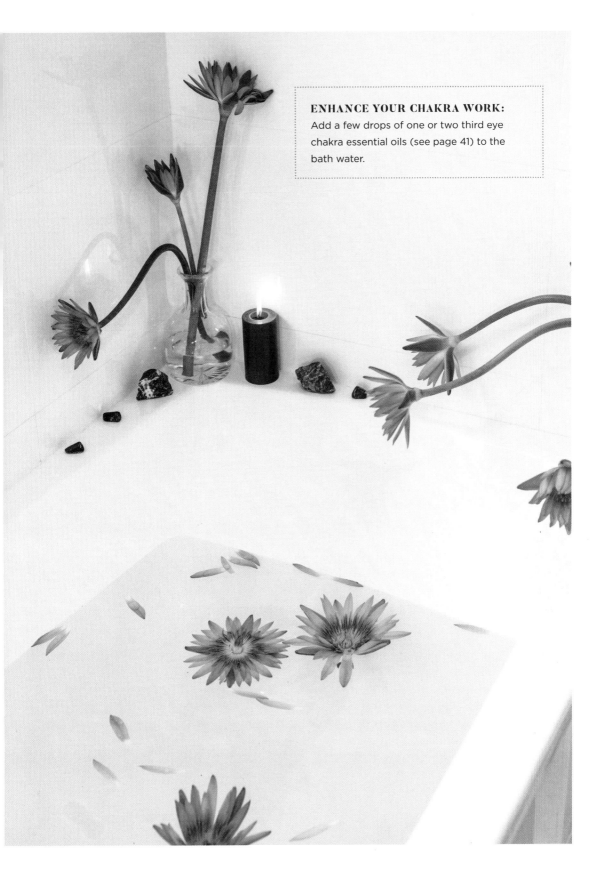

ENHANCE YOUR CHAKRA WORK:
Add a few drops of one or two third eye
chakra essential oils (see page 41) to the
bath water.

ENHANCE YOUR CHAKRA WORK:
The third eye chakra is associated with the
light element, so perform this ritual outside
at night in moonlight.

Ritual for Mindfulness

Try this ritual to bring about a calmer, wiser version of yourself. It is ideal if you
want to achieve a new state of mindful awareness.

YOU WILL NEED

- Energy cleansing toolkit (see page 50)
- Pen and paper
- One or more crystals corresponding to the third eye chakra (see page 144)
- Heatproof bowl
- Matches or lighter

METHOD

1   Find a quiet, comfortable place where you can meditate with no
    distractions. Cleanse the space, following the instructions on page 50.
2   Sit comfortably and take a few deep breaths to focus your energy and
    help you bring more intention and mindfulness into your life; this could
    include eliminating negative habits that block your intuition or commiting
    to spending more time in nature, connecting to plants and animals.
3   Write down what you would like to change in order to be in a place
    of greater connection. Add an affirmation, such as 'I am taking steps
    towards my spiritual growth' or 'I choose to live with mindfulness'.
4   Spend a couple of minutes meditating on your intentions while holding
    your crystal.
5   Focus on your third eye chakra and visualize a glowing indigo light
    expanding with each inhale. As you exhale, release any unhelpful beliefs
    relating to your consciousness and spiritual transformation. This will help
    you develop a deeper connection to your higher self.
6   To complete the process, place the piece of paper in the heatproof bowl
    and burn it, along with all you intend to release. Ensure the flames are
    fully extinguished when you are finished.

Third Eye Chakra Journaling

This seven-day exercise will help you determine the health of your third eye chakra, while allowing you to release unprocessed emotions relating to insight, perception and inner guidance. Answer one of the journal prompts below each day for a week, honouring any emotions and past experiences that come up during the process.

YOU WILL NEED
- Pen and journal

METHOD
1 Begin the exercise by sitting quietly for a few minutes, focusing on your breathing to centre your energy.
2 Pick one of the following questions and answer honestly, noticing the effect it has on you:
   - Do you trust your intuition – in what instances have you felt this?
   - Was imagination encouraged growing up, and how you can you embrace your imagination as an adult?
   - Which areas of your life do you have a strong sense of clarity about and which do you feel are unclear?
   - Are you open to learning new ideas or do you rely solely on your own beliefs?
   - When do you feel close-minded and what topics do you find most difficult to address?
   - In what ways do you have mental strength and inner wisdom, and how can you enhance this?
   - What can you do to gain a clearer vision of your life and to feel more aligned?
3 Write your responses in your journal, working through any thoughts or emotions that arise.
4 Sit for a moment and meditate on an intention to support your third eye chakra – for example, 'I am insightful and intuitive'.

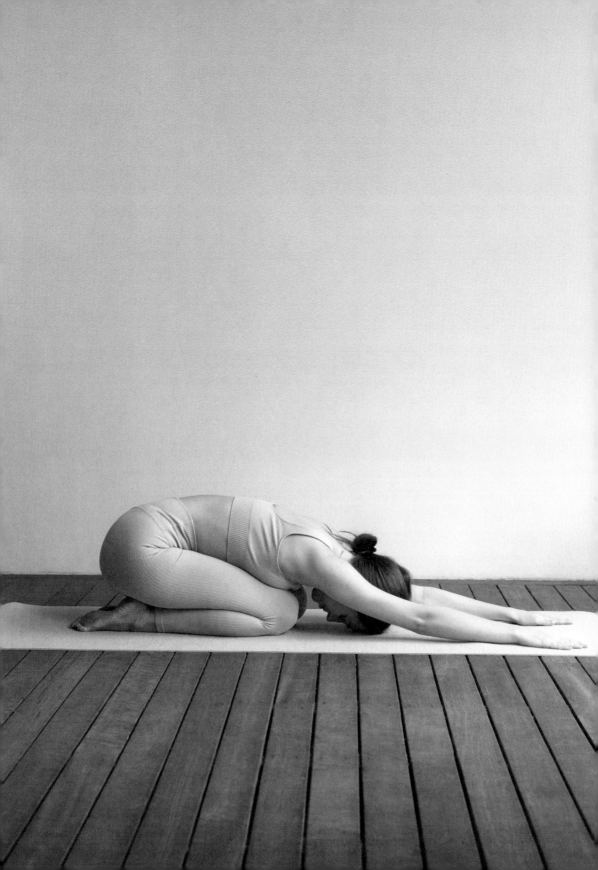

ENHANCE YOUR CHAKRA WORK:
Before you do this yoga pose, apply the
Essential Oil Blend for Clarity (see page 142)
to your wrists or over your third eye.

Yoga for Intuition

By connecting your forehead to the earth, the Extended Child's Pose
(*Balasana*) actively stimulates the third eye chakra. Try this pose to
strengthen your intuition while releasing stress and enhancing mental clarity.

YOU WILL NEED
- Comfortable, non-restrictive clothing
- Yoga mat

METHOD
1 Begin the pose in a kneeling position, adjusting your heels so that they
   rest under your hips.
2 Open your knees and walk your hands out in front of you until your arms
   are straight, or as far as you feel comfortable.
3 Spread your fingers wide and allow your forehead and arms to sink to
   the ground.
4 Allow this light pressure to bring focus to your third eye chakra and
   remain here for 3–5 breaths or longer. You may start to feel heat in this
   area or a light pulse when concentrating on this energy centre.
5 Return to your upright position to complete the exercise.

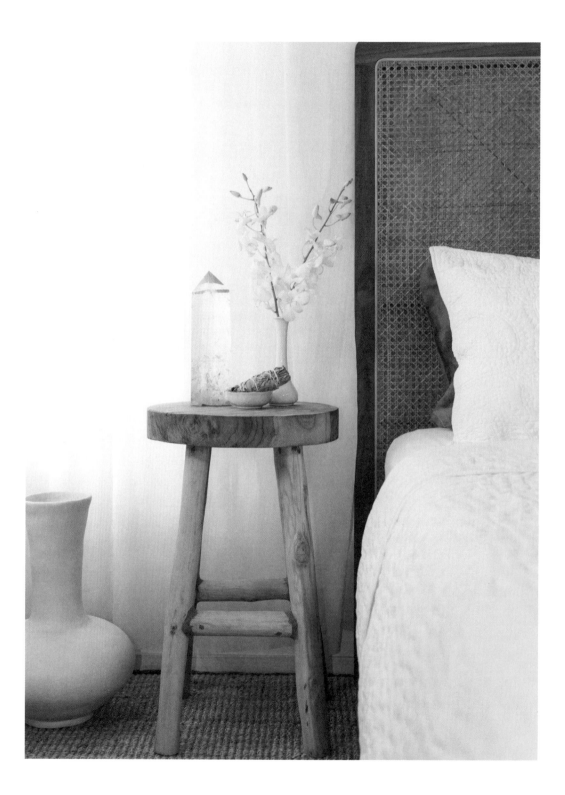

CROWN CHAKRA

SPIRITUALITY AND CONSCIOUSNESS

Tea for Divine Guidance

The crown chakra is the energy centre of spirituality and divine guidance. It corresponds to herbs and flowers carrying these mystical properties, such as lavender and tulsi leaf (holy basil). When you feel anxious or depressed, try this tea to improve mental clarity and enhance your spiritual connection to a higher power.

YOU WILL NEED (INGREDIENTS PER CUP)

- 1 teaspoon dried lavender flowers
- 1 teaspoon dried tulsi leaves
- Teapot
- 400ml (13½fl oz) boiling water
- Cup
- Sweetener of your choice (optional)

METHOD

1 Put the flowers and leaves into the teapot and pour over the boiling water.
2 Cover and leave the ingredients to steep for 5–10 minutes.
3 Pour the tea into the cup and add some sweetener, if desired.
4 Find somewhere peaceful to sit. While you drink the tea, focus on the intention of enhancing your spiritual connection.

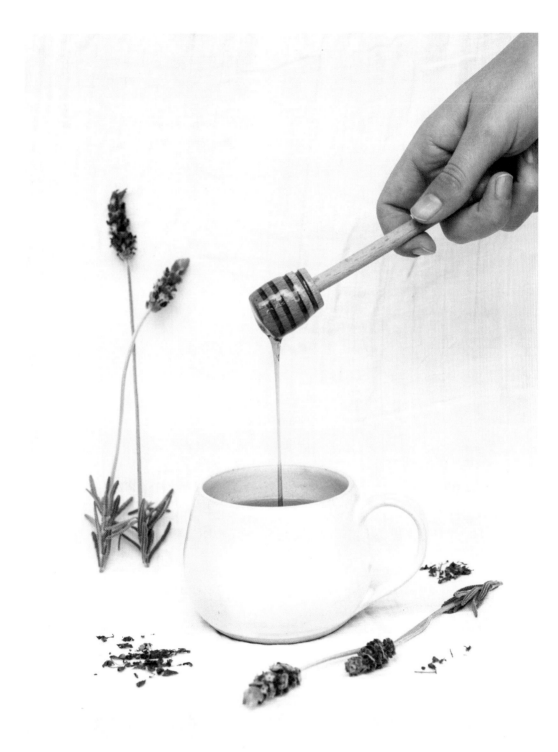

ENHANCE YOUR CHAKRA WORK:
Add a tulsi leaf or a small crown chakra
crystal (see page 160) to the bottle.

Essential Oil Blend for
Spiritual Development

Enhancing your spiritual development is an important aspect of activating the
crown chakra. When this energy centre is balanced, you feel a greater sense
of peace and trust in the universe. Use this essential oil blend to raise your
consciousness and find a sense of peace and trust in your life.

YOU WILL NEED

- 4 drops tulsi essential oil
- 12 drops pink lotus essential oil
- 4 drops lavender essential oil
- 10-ml (⅓-fl oz) glass rollerball bottle
- Small funnel or dropper
- Carrier oil, such as almond, rosehip, argan or fractionated coconut
- Blank label
- Pen

METHOD

1 Add the essential oils to the rollerball bottle.
2 Using a small funnel or dropper, top up the bottle with the carrier oil.
3 Insert the rollerball, close the lid and swirl to combine.
4 Write a label and stick it to the bottle.
5 To use the blend, roll a small amount on the inside of your wrists in a
   circular motion, or apply directly to the crown chakra to enhance your
   spiritual connection. You can also apply it before the Meditation for
   Stillness (see page 159) to enhance the practice.

ENHANCE YOUR CHAKRA WORK:
Hold a crown chakra crystal (see page 160)
in your hands during the meditation.

Meditation for Stillness

Try this exercise to create stillness when feeling overwhelmed or when your mind is overactive. This meditation is a powerful way to recentre your energy and relieve stress and tension in the face of burnout.

YOU WILL NEED

- Oil burner or diffuser
- Matches or lighter
- One or more crown chakra essential oils (see page 45)

METHOD

1 Find a quiet, comfortable place where you can meditate with no distractions. Light the oil burner or diffuser and add the essential oils.

2 Sit in a comfortable position, with your spine straight and your shoulders relaxed. Close your eyes and take a few deep breaths, allowing your mind and body to relax completely. Feel the tension release from your face, jaw, neck and shoulders right down to your toes.

3 Now bring your focus to your crown chakra, taking note of any feelings that arise. Do you feel connected to the spirit realms? Do you feel a sense of spiritual awareness? Focus on feeling present in your body. Don't worry if your mind wanders; just gently bring your attention back to your breathing.

4 Visualize a bright violet light where your crown chakra resides. Imagine this glowing ball of light growing brighter with each inhale.

5 As you exhale, focus on calming your mind and opening yourself up to your inner guidance as you begin to experience a sense of peace and acceptance. Feel the aroma of essential oils fill every cell in your body.

6 When you are ready to open your eyes, take a few deep breaths and experience a deep sense of openness, before bringing your awareness back to your surroundings.

7 Turn off the burner or diffuser.

Stones for Balancing
the Crown Chakra

As this chakra is responsible for spiritual awareness and divine guidance, it is supported by crystals and gemstones that carry healing properties of spirituality, expansion and enlightenment. Use these crystals to strengthen your crown chakra energy and expand your consciousness.

Moonstone

Moonstone enhances both spiritual and personal growth. It boosts emotional awareness and heightens intuition, while protecting against negative forces.

HOW TO USE THIS STONE
Carry moonstone to quieten the mind and maintain an open state of awareness.

Selenite

A stone of deep inner peace and light, selenite carries a calming energy that is beneficial in healing the crown chakra. It brings deeper understanding and expands consciousness while clearing negative energy.

HOW TO USE THIS STONE
Place selenite under your pillow to strengthen your crown chakra and remove stagnant energy while you sleep.

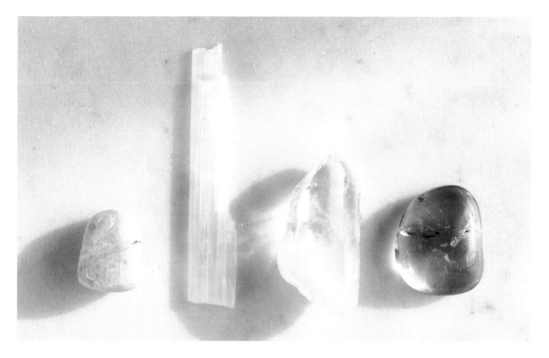

From left to right: moonstone, selenite, clear quartz and amethyst.

Clear Quartz

Believed to be the most powerful energy amplifier on this earth, clear quartz carries a high spiritual vibration. It promotes personal growth and spiritual transformation while purifying its surrounding energy.

HOW TO USE THIS STONE
Place over the crown chakra during meditation to detoxify your energy.

Amethyst

This stone carries a range of healing powers relating to both the third eye and crown chakras. It cleanses and purifies the higher energy centres to provide mental clarity and relief from anxiety, while strengthening spiritual awareness.

HOW TO USE THIS STONE
Wear amethyst to calm the mind and enhance knowledge of the spiritual realm.

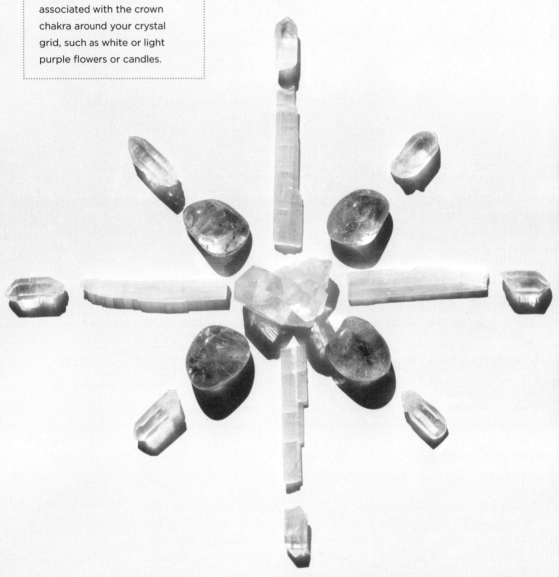

Crystal Grid for Peace and Acceptance

The stones selected for this grid carry high spiritual vibrations that promote divine guidance, insight, connection and higher knowing. Try this exercise when going through a difficult experience, to help develop a sense of peace and acceptance.

YOU WILL NEED

- A clean flat surface
- Energy cleansing toolkit (see page 50)
- 1 clear quartz
- 4 selenite
- 4 amethyst (or moonstone)
- 8 more clear quartz

METHOD

1. Decide on a flat surface to keep your grid; this should be on a table or shelf that you can revisit, but which won't be in the way of your everyday life.
2. Cleanse the crystals and the space, following the instructions on page 50.
3. Set your intention for the grid, giving the crystals a specific purpose – for example, 'I trust in divine guidance' or 'I am connected to the universe'.
4. Begin creating your grid, starting with the main centre crystal; in this case, a clear quartz.
5. Add the four selenite stones, placing one on each side of the clear quartz.
6. Place your four amethyst crystals (or moonstone) in between the selenite.
7. Now place the remaining clear quartz crystals around the outside of the other stones to form a symmetrical pattern.
8. Complete the process by focusing your energy on your intention for a minute or two. Visualize yourself feeling full of light and divine guidance.
9. Leave your grid in place for as long as you like, remembering to cleanse it occasionally and to refocus your intention.

Bath for Connecting to the Universe

This peaceful bathing ritual uses crown chakra elements, such as pink lotus or lavender, moonstone crystals and white or violet candles, to heighten your spiritual awareness and connect to your seventh energy centre. Find comfort in this exercise when going through a major shift in life, or when you simply feel disconnected from yourself or the universe.

YOU WILL NEED
- Energy cleansing toolkit (see page 50)
- Crown chakra crystals (see page 160); note that selenite and moonstone should be placed around the bath and not immersed in water
- Sea salt or Epsom salts for extra cleansing and relaxation
- Crown chakra flowers (see page 45)
- Lavender or tulsi tea
- White or violet beeswax or soy candles
- Calming music

METHOD
1. Cleanse the bathroom, following the instructions on page 50.
2. Run the bath, slowly adding in your healing crystals, bath salts and flowers. Add the herbal tea directly to your bath water, or save it to sip while you are bathing. Light your candles and play calming music to create a peaceful atmosphere.
3. Once you are comfortably in the bath, focus on your breathing. Close your eyes and visualize your crown chakra as a bright spinning wheel of energy.
4. Let go of any tension in your body as you begin to feel centred. Choose an affirmation or intention relating to your seventh chakra – for example, 'I am at peace' or 'I trust in the universe' – to meditate on as you attract new meaning into your life.
5. Extinguish the candles safely.
6. Enjoy moving further into your spiritual power.

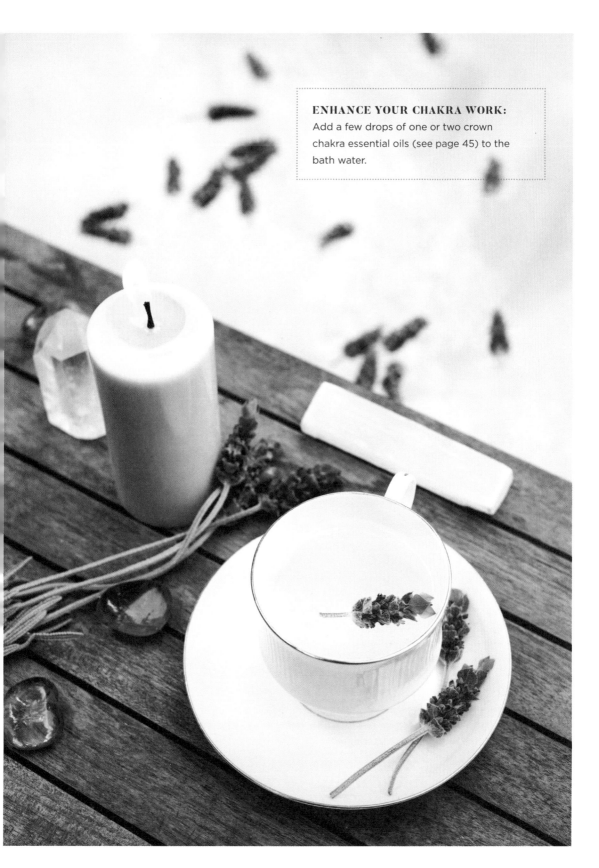

ENHANCE YOUR CHAKRA WORK:
Add a few drops of one or two crown
chakra essential oils (see page 45) to the
bath water.

Ritual for Self-transformation

Try this ritual if there are changes you would like to make in your life; allow
this exercise to guide you in the right direction.

YOU WILL NEED

- Energy cleansing toolkit (see page 50)
- Pen and paper
- One or more crystals corresponding to the crown chakra (see page 160)
- Heatproof bowl
- Matches or lighter

METHOD

1. Find a quiet, comfortable place where you can meditate with no
   distractions. Cleanse the space, following the instructions on page 50.
2. Sit comfortably and take a few deep breaths to focus your energy. Think
   about how you would like to grow and expand. What energy do you wish
   to call in to help you live in a more peaceful, aware state?
3. Write down what you would like to change in order to live from a place
   of growth and connection. Add an affirmation, such as 'I seek positive
   experiences that nourish my spirit'.
4. Spend a few minutes meditating on your intentions while holding your crystal.
5. Focus on your crown chakra and visualize a glowing violet light
   expanding with each inhale. As you exhale, release any unhelpful beliefs
   relating to your personal growth and transformation. This will help you
   develop a deeper connection to your higher self and will allow you to feel
   more present, accepting and at peace.
6. To complete the process, place the piece of paper in the heatproof bowl
   and burn it, along with all you intend to release. Ensure the flames are
   fully extinguished when you are finished.

Crown Chakra Journaling

This seven-day exercise will help you determine the health of your crown chakra, while enabling you to release unprocessed emotions relating to your spiritual development. Answer one of the journal prompts below each day for a week, honouring any emotions and past experiences that come up during the process.

YOU WILL NEED
- Pen and journal

METHOD
1 Begin the exercise by sitting quietly for a few minutes, focusing on your breathing to centre your energy.
2 Pick one of the following questions and answer honestly, noticing the effect it has on you:
   - Do you have a sense of spiritual awareness, and what does spirituality mean to you?
   - Do you trust in the universe or do you find it difficult to have faith in this area of your life?
   - What can you do to prioritize self-growth and reflection?
   - Are you able to practise patience and stillness or do you find it difficult to be at peace?
   - How would you describe your outlook on life – do you feel you are where you are meant to be?
   - Would you describe yourself as someone who lives in the present moment or are you often looking too far into your past or your future?
   - What can you do to create a greater connection to your higher self?
3 Write your responses in your journal, working through any thoughts or emotions that arise.
4 Sit for a moment and meditate on an intention to support your crown chakra – for example, 'I am at peace'.

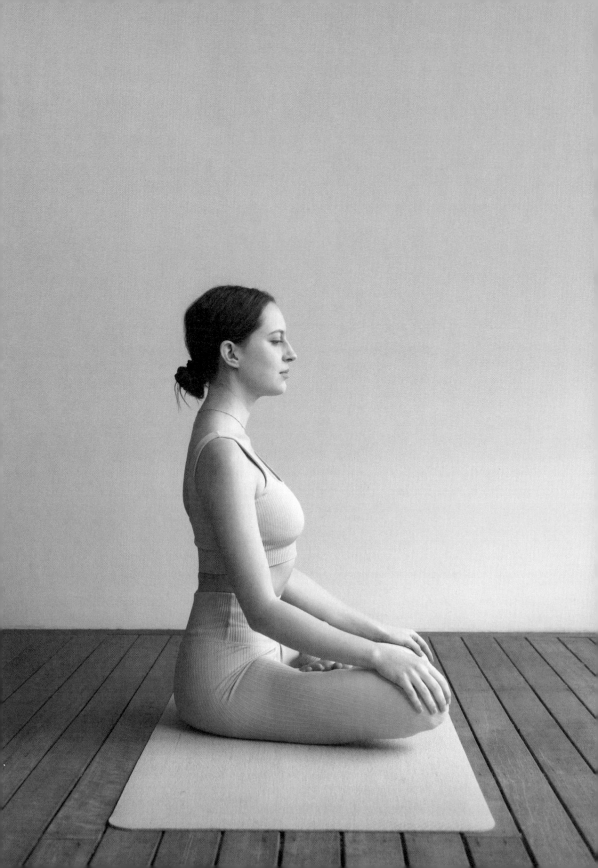

ENHANCE YOUR CHAKRA WORK:
Before you do this yoga pose, apply the
Essential Oil Blend for Spiritual Development
(see page 158) to your wrists or over your
crown chakra.

Yoga for Spiritual Connection

The seventh chakra represents the 'thousand-petalled lotus' and is the centre
of our spirituality and higher awareness. Try Lotus Pose (*Padmasana*) to
access your divine consciousness and to develop your spiritual connection
in times of uncertainty.

YOU WILL NEED
- Comfortable, non-restrictive clothing
- Yoga mat

METHOD
1   Begin the pose in a seated position on the ground, placing a foot on each
    of your thighs. If you are more comfortable in the Half Lotus pose, you
    can position just one foot on your thigh, resting the other on the floor.
2   Rest your hands on your knees and keep your posture straight
    but relaxed.
3   Lower your gaze or close your eyes, taking 3–5 breaths to calm
    your mind.
4   Bring your awareness to your crown chakra and spend as much time here
    as you like.

Index of Fixes by Need

General Index

Acknowledgements

I would like to acknowledge and thank the people in my life for their encouragement and support during the writing of this book. Each of you has played an important role through this process and I am so grateful to you all.

Bali Benson, my best friend and fiancé, for always bringing such joy and light. Thank you for inspiring me each day and for keeping me grounded and present.

Mallika Des Fours, my mother, for her kind, caring and generous spirit, which has taught me to live with purpose and grace. Thank you for all that you do for me.

Dhyana Thornbury, my sister, for always encouraging and supporting my projects. Thank you for working alongside me to keep Luminosity Crystals growing and expanding.

James Thornbury, my father, for his spiritual presence, which has continued to guide and support me long after his passing. Thank you for teaching me to live with gratitude and intention.

The White Lion publishing team, for their hard work, expertise and dedication to this project. Thank you for giving me the opportunity to make this book a reality – I am forever grateful.

About the Author

Australian author and business owner Juliette Thornbury is a certified crystal healer and energy worker. She is the creator of Luminosity Crystals, a thriving online business that is renowned for its sustainable and high-quality sourcing. Author of the best-selling book *The Crystal Fix*, Juliette has worked with different forms of energy healing to assist clients all around the world. Follow Juliette on Instagram @luminositycrystals.